The Gut Flush Plan

*The Breakthrough Cleansing Program
to Rid Your Body of the Toxins
That Make You Sick,
Tired, and Bloated*

ANN LOUISE GITTLEMAN, PH.D., CNS

AVERY
A MEMBER OF
PENGUIN GROUP (USA) INC.
NEW YORK

AVERY

Published by the Penguin Group
Penguin Group (USA) Inc., 375 Hudson Street, New York, New York 10014, USA •
Penguin Group (Canada), 90 Eglinton Avenue East, Suite 700, Toronto, Ontario
M4P 2Y3, Canada (a division of Pearson Canada Inc.) • Penguin Books Ltd,
80 Strand, London WC2R 0RL, England • Penguin Ireland, 25 St Stephen's Green,
Dublin 2, Ireland (a division of Penguin Books Ltd) • Penguin Group (Australia),
250 Camberwell Road, Camberwell, Victoria 3124, Australia (a division of Pearson
Australia Group Pty Ltd) • Penguin Books India Pvt Ltd, 11 Community Centre,
Panchsheel Park, New Delhi–110 017, India • Penguin Group (NZ), 67 Apollo Drive,
Rosedale, North Shore 0632, New Zealand (a division of Pearson New Zealand Ltd) •
Penguin Books (South Africa) (Pty) Ltd, 24 Sturdee Avenue,
Rosebank, Johannesburg 2196, South Africa

Penguin Books Ltd, Registered Offices: 80 Strand, London WC2R 0RL, England

Most Avery books are available at special quantity discounts for bulk purchase for sales promotions, premiums, fund-
raising, and educational needs. Special books or book excerpts also can be created to fit specific needs. For details, write
Penguin Group (USA) Inc. Special Markets, 375 Hudson Street, New York, NY 10014.

Library of Congress Cataloging-in-Publication Data

Gittleman, Ann Louise.
The gut flush plan : the breakthrough cleansing program to rid your body of the toxins that make you sick, tired, and
bloated / Ann Louise Gittleman.
p.   cm.
Includes bibliographical references and index.
ISBN 978-1-58333-309-9
1. Detoxification (Health).   2. Colon (Anatomy).   I. Title.
RA784.5.G582   2008   2008006370
612.3—dc22

Printed in the United States of America
1   3   5   7   9   10   8   6   4   2

BOOK DESIGN BY TANYA MAIBORODA

Neither the publisher nor the author is engaged in rendering professional advice or services to the individual reader. The
ideas, procedures, and suggestions contained in this book are not intended as a substitute for consulting with your physician. All matters regarding your health require medical supervision. Neither the author nor the publisher shall be liable or
responsible for any loss or damage allegedly arising from any information or suggestion in this book.

The recipes contained in this book are to be followed exactly as written. The publisher is not responsible for your specific
health or allergy needs that may require medical supervision. The publisher is not responsible for any adverse reactions to
the recipes contained in this book.

While the author has made every effort to provide accurate telephone numbers and Internet addresses at the time of publication, neither the publisher nor the author assumes any responsibility for errors, or for changes that occur after publication. Further, the publisher does not have any control over and does not assume any responsibility for author or
third-party websites or their content.

The
Gut Flush
Plan

Acknowledgments

THIS BOOK IS TRULY AN EXAMPLE OF ART IMITATING LIFE. THROUGH A mysterious sequence of events, I had the opportunity, during the writing of this book, to experience just about all the ailments I write about. Needless to say, it provided me with a newfound respect and admiration for all the people I met and consulted with who are in some degree of daily pain from gut-related issues.

I am very grateful to my publisher, Megan Newman, for seeing the need for a book like this and for inspiring the entire Avery team to make it a reality and a passion. My profound thanks go to Miriam Rich, assistant editor; to Ann Kosmoski, publicity manager; and to Amanda Tobier, marketing director, for being on top of all the related news articles and publicity.

As always, I am very indebted to my literary agent, Coleen O'Shea, who has been a staunch advocate of the topic and of my thirty books in general. Coleen encouraged, cajoled, and persisted in making me see "the light" when I was feeling "out of sorts" because of my own gut-flush saga during the writing of this book.

Mariska van Aalst was the creative force behind much of the book's organization and creative punch. She is an angel to work with, and I would welcome the opportunity to work with her again. Carl Lowe provided lots of cutting-edge research, which was very helpful and relevant to the topic, while Karen Jarmon lent a helping hand in "directing" operations for a while. Our wonderful recipes and menu plans came from my own personal chef, Pamela Wright. Linda Sue Shapiro later lent her most capable and professional expertise in testing all the Gut Flush recipes in her professional Gut Flush kitchen and in tweaking menus, recipes, and shopping lists for publication.

Kudos to my personal team of supporters on the home front: to James William Templeton, for everything in every way; to Pamela Wright, who fed me the most wonderfully nutritious and delicious meals à la Gut Flush; to my team of chiropractors, who kept my head on straight from coast to coast: Dr. Natalie Engelbart, Dr. Brad Reed, Dr. Paul Schutz, Dr. Allan Joubert, and Dr. Roy Speiser; to my bodyworkers, Laura Evenson, Marjanna Ylitalo, and Leslie Mulvihill; to my naturopathic associates, Dr. Roger Rowse and Dr. Bruce Blinzler; to my local dentists, Dr. Armand DeFelice and Dr. Robert Stephan; to my dear colonic therapists, Kathie Moe, Lolyn Pobram, and Georgia Cold; to my invaluable office staff: Stuart Gittleman, director of operations and business manager; Tami Oliver, personal assistant; moderators Linda Sue Shapiro, Carol Ackerman, Janine Forbes, Sue Durand, Cathy Young, Mandy Troxell, Linda Pankhurst, Jackie Scott, Charli Sorenson, Michelle O., and Nina Moreau; and my amazing Web guru, Amelia Kleymann.

My most sincere thanks to Dr. Hal Huggins, Dr. Stuart Nunnally, Dr. Lane Freeman, and the entire staff at Healthy Smiles for Life for making me realize that it really was "all in my head" after all!

Finally, I wish to thank my readers and professional associates for allowing me the time to reflect and create this work. My blessings and thanks to everyone.

To the millions of GI sufferers, who I pray will be encouraged to take "the road less traveled" because of this book.

Contents

Introduction:
Food Fright

TODAY, MORE THAN EVER BEFORE, OUR BODIES ARE BOMBARDED BY chemicals, environmental pollutants, nasty bacteria, and parasites. These toxins can spread far beyond the digestive tract and, in some cases, turn deadly. Even the produce aisle, where fruits and veggies had always been a safe haven for health-conscious and calorie-concerned consumers, is getting scary. You know what I mean because practically every day, we see headlines like these:

Melamine in Pet Food . . .
Salmonella Contaminates Peanut Butter in 26 States . . .
Bagged Spinach Tainted by E. coli . . .
Contaminated Beef Recalled in 22 States . . .
The Parasite Cryptosporidium Survives Chlorination and May Contaminate Tap Water . . .
Parasite in Tap Water May Cause Blindness . . .

It's enough to make you feel queasy and never want to drink straight from the tap again.

Dodging dangers at the dinner table seems to be a full-time job nowadays.

And as a professional nutritionist and author of thirty books on health and healing, I'm not just worried by the disturbing trends in food safety, I'm downright alarmed. I have been in the health care field for more than three decades and I can't recall a time when I've seen more people suffer with so many problems related to food.

And, recently, I became one of them.

I thought I had been doing everything "right," following my own protective protocols, taking daily probiotics and digestive enzymes. Yet, for months, I suffered from bloating, abdominal cramping, embarrassing gas, and anxiety. After several trips to Urgent Care, I was "diagnosed" with acid reflux based on my symptoms. I then decided to try every natural remedy I was familiar with for heartburn, GERD, and digestive ills—all to no avail.

I became so desperate that I resorted to commonly prescribed medications like Protonix, Prevacid, and Nexium, which only made me feel worse and very disoriented. When an upper GI scope showed that I was "as clean as a whistle," I was even more upset. Here I was, the "First Lady of Nutrition," not knowing what was going on in my body and finding no answers. I was sick, suffering, and stymied.

After six full months of major discomfort, I decided to follow the advice that I would normally have given to a client or a reader who presented the same baffling array of symptoms that I was experiencing: I did a stool test. Finally, I was able to get to the root cause of what was really going on in my body.

My expanded GI panel stool analysis revealed that I was harboring abundant Candida albicans and rarified yeast, abundant inflammatory bacteria with exotic names like Klebsiella and Citrobacter species as well as some rare alpha-hemolytic Streptococcus. Not your ordinary bacteria, by any means. So how did I, of all people, manage to "pick up" all of these bugs? You will be shocked to find out—it may be something you do every day but don't really think about how you put your body at risk.

I'll talk more about this experience later in the book, but I share this story now to let you know that we are truly all in this together. This experience was one of the inspirations behind the development of *The Gut Flush Plan*. I am deeply concerned about unsafe food handling and the dangers in our food supply and in our environment. With this book and this plan, I want to prevent what happened to me from happening to you.

We are supposed to have the safest food and water supply in the world, but as a nation we seem to be sick and getting sicker with every meal. The Centers for Disease Control and Prevention (CDC) report that more than two hundred thousand Americans get food poisoning every single day. On a yearly basis, almost 80 million of us get sick, and more than three hundred thousand go to the hospital, for food-related illness. And these are just the unfortunate victims we know about. Many more people may actually be contracting food-borne illnesses and simply don't realize their food and drink could be making them ill.

Worse still, we're importing the problem at an increasing rate. In the first four months of 2007, the Food and Drug Administration (FDA) seized about three hundred food shipments from China. The seafood, candy, and other items had been contaminated with chemicals such as pesticides, antibiotics, antifungals, and formaldehyde. But despite all the problems with imports, the FDA, hampered by personnel and budget constraints, inspects only about *one percent* of the $60 billion of imported food each year.

Frightened yet? Me, too, and with good reason.

You and I are not being paranoid. The sources of our food are increasingly out of our hands. When giant conglomerates mass-produce assembly lines full of processed food, supermarket chains import food of questionable origin from all over the world, and corporate farmers grow vegetables in polluted environments, we're right to question the safety of the food on our forks.

And while the food supply has gotten scarier, our digestive systems have also become weaker and less capable of coping with food-related upsets. We spend more than $60 billion every year for medical help for our digestive problems, which are now the second most common reason for visits to physicians. (I can't even begin to tell you how many people consult me because their digestion is "off.")

You've heard of the new types of bacteria—the "Superbugs"—that are quickly spreading through hospitals, gyms, schools, beauty salons, and the community? A recent report in the *Journal of the American Medical Association* found that more than nineteen thousand deaths a year can be attributed to MRSA, or methicillin-resistant Staphylococcus aureus, a type of Superbug once found exclusively in hospitals that has now leaked into community settings. Among other things, the massive amounts of antibiotics force-fed to conventional livestock have contributed to a dangerous antibiotic resistance that has allowed these Superbugs to thrive. And our weakened digestive systems have only helped make us sitting ducks for their deadly infections.

The fact is, due to certain diet and lifestyle habits we've developed—from mindlessly munching on our favorite corn chips to compulsively using antibacterial soaps—we've become part of the problem. We've made ourselves susceptible to a wide range of food-related challenges, ranging from the more common occurrences like food sensitivities and stomachaches to more serious, long-term manifestations such as irritable bowel syndrome, spastic colon, severe constipation, ulcerative colitis, and Crohn's disease. We're a nation suffering from a raging case of what I call Gut Grief.

I know we can fight back. Thus far, amidst all the headlines that scream, the *real* news has been absent from the front pages. And here it is: you *can* take concrete steps right now, today, to protect yourself. You can stand up against the invasion of pathogens, parasites, and other undesirables in your food that seek to camp out in your belly and make you sick. Just a simple set of practical, concrete steps can dramatically lower your risk of getting sick—and may even save your life.

I've spent my entire career helping people identify and pinpoint the "hidden invaders" or unsuspected factors that may be sabotaging their health. For many years, I have seen my patients recover from unresolved illnesses after getting rid of parasites. Their ailments had been mislabeled as depression, allergies, hypoglycemia, chronic fatigue syndrome, or even fibromyalgia. As I took their history, I would always ask about recent travel, for instance. A camping trip in the wilderness or a visit to Mexico, Asia, or a tropical island frequently preceded persistent flulike symptoms, extreme tiredness, intermittent diarrhea and constipation, or even sudden weight loss or weight gain. The connection between parasites and your health is well documented in my book *Guess What Came to Dinner?* which I updated in 2001 to reflect how a number of factors (travel, the increasing contamination of municipal and rural water supplies, day-care centers, increasing popularity of exotic regional foods, and the continued popularity of household pets) have continued to contribute to the silent parasite epidemic I believe we experience today.

Similarly, in my book *The Fat Flush Plan* I discuss the neglected and overlooked weight gain factors, beyond just diet and exercise, that are major contributors to our current obesity epidemic that has claimed seven out of ten Americans. In the Fat Flush Plan, I target liver toxicity, waterlogged tissues, the fear of eating fat, excess insulin/excess inflammation, and stress as potent factors that are "weighing us down."

Now I have turned my attention to the multiple factors that threaten our poor ailing guts. Given my own puzzling gut-related case history coupled with the rising tides of tainted foods, Superbugs, and other scary headlines, I knew it was time to develop a program that could protect against this new breed of twenty-first-century ills. Enter *The Gut Flush Plan.*

Recent science has shown us, beyond a shadow of a doubt, that food, digestion, and health are inextricably linked. In this book, you will learn surprising new information about how nutritious meals can "rebuild" a digestive system that efficiently absorbs nutrients, eliminates toxins, and helps the immune system protect the body from invading pathogens.

We'll begin by discussing the very real dangers that lurk both around the world and in your refrigerator, whether the "bad bugs" can give you a short-term case of food poisoning or the more dangerous strains can cause long-term illness or turn downright deadly.

Then we'll consider your individual symptoms: Do you suffer from recurring diarrhea? Chronic constipation? Irritable bowel? Acid reflux? We'll use those symptoms to determine your greatest risks: Are you overrun with yeast? Do you harbor an unknown parasite? Have you adopted an antibiotic-resistant Superbug? Are you sensitive to certain foods, without knowing which ones?

We'll talk about how each of these conditions is contracted, how and why they are on the rise, and what you can do about them. You'll take a self-diagnostic quiz to determine your level of risk, so you can follow a protocol specially designed to prevent and relieve each one.

Once you're on the road to relieving your most pressing intestinal issues, you'll turn to the core of *The Gut Flush Plan,* the Gut Flush eating and supplement program. Designed to help everyone defend themselves against yeast, Superbugs, parasites, food sensitivities, and other food-borne illnesses, the Gut Flush eating and supplement program is a revolutionary three-step process to rebuild your digestive system from a cellular level up. You will learn to:

- **Fortify** your own compromised digestive system against pathogens and parasites;
- **Flush** out any lingering infestations or toxicities;
- **Feed** yourself nourishing foods that encourage gut health and don't trigger sensitivities.

The preventative steps and therapeutic solutions in this eating and lifestyle program feature all the knowledge, tips, and techniques you'll ever need to free yourself from Gut Grief and keep you and your family safe from food-borne illness. You'll learn how to defend yourself against tainted foods, even name brands that you have come to trust. You'll find out which mealtime staples undermine your best efforts at weight control by feeding greedy parasites or triggering food sensitivities and bloat. You'll discover how to naturally boost your body's production of beneficial intestinal flora (also known as probiotics), hydrochloric acid (HCl), and digestive enzymes, your three greatest allies in the fight against Gut Grief. You will also learn that safe food handling is the most neglected subject in food preparation but perhaps the most important of all. As you go, you'll savor delicious new foods and discover tweaks to your favorite dishes that can make them your strongest allies in the fight to enhance immunity and reduce intestinal distress.

Best of all, *The Gut Flush Plan* will give you the power to feel in control of your own health, both now and in the future. Enter into the plan and, among many other benefits, you can expect to:

- regain your energy and vitality by eradicating pathogenic bacteria, parasites, yeast, and food allergies;
- enhance healthy bowel function by establishing regular, pain-free bowel movements;
- increase your production of critical, health-protecting vitamins, such as the B vitamins and vitamin K;
- soothe agonizing maladies, such as peptic ulcers, acid reflux, and heartburn;
- relieve embarrassing bloating and gas;
- cleanse toxic, undigested food from your colon and lower intestine;

- help control irritable bowel syndrome, Crohn's disease, diverticulitis, celiac disease, and spastic colon;
- enhance your overall immunity;
- lose stubborn, unwanted pounds.

Food-related problems are everywhere and show no signs of going away. But you don't have to be a victim. You can be a person who feels lighter, cleaner, healthier, and more vital. You can face the twenty-first-century food supply without fear and once again delight in the simple pleasure of eating deliciously clean and safe foods. Begin the Gut Flush Plan and start living today.

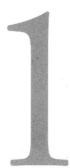

Why You Need the Gut Flush Plan

1

You *Can* Fight Gut Grief

MY FRIEND MARTY JEAN IS A HUGE FAN OF PEANUT BUTTER. ONE NIGHT, after enjoying a late-night peanut butter sandwich before bed, she awoke with horrific pains in her stomach. She was gripped by an overwhelming nausea and felt like she might pass out from the excruciating cramps in her gut.

She stumbled through the dark house into the kitchen and headed straight for her vitamin cabinet. That's where she kept her stash of a revolutionary probiotic, a supplement containing multiple strains of viable lactic acid bacteria that was formulated by an award-winning Japanese microbiologist. Marty Jean knew that these probiotics contained a new bacterial strain proven to neutralize a wide scope of resistant microorganisms, and somehow, in her painful fog, she realized she was in the grips of a particularly virulent strain. She'd heard about this particular type of probiotics helping people in her situation and she prayed they would help relieve her pain. She systematically chewed one capsule after another—ten in total—and crawled her way to the bathroom to wait out the rest of the attack.

After sweating it out for about twenty minutes, Marty Jean felt the cramps and urge to vomit slowly pass. With tremendous relief, she was able to move her bowels. She washed her hands and face, rinsed out her mouth, and slipped back under the covers, desperate for sleep.

In the morning when she woke up, it took her a minute to remember what had happened the night before. She had no cramps, no gas, no nothing. She got up and took a shower, silently marveling at her experience. Before she'd taken the probiotics, she'd been trying to decide whom to wake up to take her to the emergency room. But instead, she'd finished out the night in a very peaceful sleep.

While she prepared her breakfast, she turned on the morning news. One of the lead stories was about her favorite brand of peanut butter. Indeed, as she had suspected, her beloved snack was the culprit behind her middle-of-the-night stomach woes, which in fact was an acute case of Salmonella poisoning. Marty Jean was lucky—she knew what to do—unlike the hundreds of people who also got sick, with more than fifty ending up in the hospital. Her special probiotics had helped her fight back.

None of us wants to think about what frightening food pathogen may be lurking in our next meal. Unfortunately, we must. We live in a world with rising numbers of Superbugs like Salmonella and E. coli. Without proper regulations in place, questionable food handling practices will carry on, unabated. And something tells me large food corporations will continue to take shortcuts with quality and safety in favor of profit.

Unless we take action to protect ourselves, we are all sitting ducks for Gut Grief.

Nearly one thousand people a day are rushed to the hospital because of something they ate. But you don't have to be one of them. When you follow the Gut Flush Plan, you can tap into the health defenses Mother Nature designed for you.

We are all born with solid armor for this food battle, and these natural defenses are formidable. We just have to be attentive, learn a few strategies, and follow the natural ways to restore balance in our intestinal tract. We have to learn to Fortify, Flush, and Feed our digestive systems with the foods and supplements that allow them to work the way nature intended.

While everyone who lives in a world of compromised food safety and imbalanced bacteria can benefit from the core Gut Flush Plan, some of us may be suffering from more Gut Grief than others. Let's look at some of the painful and uncomfortable Gut Grief symptoms that may have drawn you to this book.

When a Good Gut Goes Bad

A toxic colon is a major factor in the development of seemingly unrelated symptoms that extend far beyond the GI tract. If any of these conditions represent your chief health complaint, it may be a sign that your gut is indeed the cause of your grief:

- ulcers
- food sensitivities
- disrupted sleep
- digestive difficulties
- yeast infections
- frequent cold and respiratory infections
- persistent aches and pains
- bad breath
- gum infections
- irritable bowel syndrome
- diarrhea
- constipation
- chronic fatigue
- unexplained weight loss or gain
- skin problems like acne, eczema, and psoriasis
- arthritis and other inflammatory problems
- painful menstruation
- menopausal discomforts

When you Fortify, Flush, and Feed your gut, you'll start on the right track to rid yourself of these problems. In Chapter 2, we'll talk about four of the main sources of these complaints: yeast overgrowth, parasite infestation, Superbug attacks, and food sensitivities. But first, let's look at a few of the most common symptoms of Gut Grief, among the dozens of others we'll discuss throughout the book.

Disruptive Digestion

We all want our meals to be satisfying and have a little staying power—but we also want the food to *leave* our bodies at a certain point. After you eat, your meal should stay in your digestive system for only twelve to eighteen hours before either being absorbed or eliminated as fecal matter. This transit time allows toxins to be ousted before they can do you any harm.

Twelve to eighteen hours is the ideal, but in today's world of fast food, trans fats, sugar, fiberless diets, pharmaceuticals, and over-the-counter drugs, most people's colons have been trained to hold onto these waste products for *two to seven days.* Talk about a clogged byway! You wouldn't want to dip your hand into toxic waste and hold it there for an entire week. But when your digestion is lethargic and your stool hangs around your colon longer than it should, your colon wall endures just that kind of exposure due to putrefying and rotting wastes that create autointoxication (or self-poisoning).

This toxic environment in the bowel then makes the bowel too alkaline to inhibit the growth of pathogens. It will also kill off the beneficial bacteria—also known as probiotics—that live in the lining of the intestines, which require an acidic pH environment of about 5.5 to 6.5 to thrive and adhere. (I'll talk extensively about these beneficial bacteria, one of Mother Nature's most impressive defenses—as well as the importance of the colon-sweeping insoluble fiber and soluble fiber, the "real" super food that feeds these beneficial bacteria and nourishes the colon's cells—throughout the book, starting on page 19 [see "Probiotics, the *Good* Bacteria" in Chapter 2].)

To function properly, the colon constantly produces mucus that helps move the waste products in our feces. When the colon is irritated by stress, medications, or food intolerances, or even parasites or worms, it produces extra mucus in an effort to defend its sensitive lining. However, despite the extra mucus, irritation and inflammation always lead to breaks in the mucous barrier. That allows bacteria and parasites to hide under a protective covering of mucus and often causes persistent infection, a cycle that keeps repeating itself as the irritation and inflammation continue. The Gut Flush Plan allows you to Fortify, Flush, and Feed the colon so it can calm down and redirect its attention back to protecting our optimal health, instead of constantly reacting to these chronic irritations.

Constipation

Widespread constipation is one of the surest signs that America's colons are malfunctioning. Today, two out of three people over age sixty-five use laxatives. We spend upward of $1.2 *billion* a year on laxatives. Can you imagine? What a tremendous amount of money spent on a symptom that can often be easily remedied with changes in diet and exercise habits.

The trouble is, constipation goes beyond being uncomfortable—it can spell danger. Your bowel movements don't just relieve you of harmless waste—they rid your body of potentially harmful toxins, too.

At the risk of sounding anal, let's get specific: if your colon functioned at optimal capacity, you would have an easy bowel movement three times a day, about an hour or two after every meal. The color would be medium brown with the consistency of toothpaste. The stool would be approximately eight to twelve inches long with little or no odor. There would be little residue on the toilet paper, and this ideal bowel movement would leave your body effortlessly, without straining.

To put this more scientifically, you would experience the gastrocolic reflex that almost effortlessly empties the bowel. Nerves in the stomach would recognize the ingestion of food; the colon muscles would tighten and expel waste. You would let it happen, not force it, and you wouldn't have to push to make it happen.

If this doesn't sound like you, and you have fewer than two or three bowel movements a day, you may be constipated. In today's world, many things interfere with your normal, natural digestion and cause constipation:

- Nearly 50 percent of chronic constipation is caused or made worse by medications. The most common offenders are antidepressants, pain meds, and iron supplements.
- A sedentary lifestyle contributes to flaccid colon contractions. Couch potatoes have recalcitrant colons.
- Laxatives, tobacco, and caffeine (especially from coffee) irritate the colon and leave the muscles unresponsive and weak. Caffeine, a kind of stimulant laxative, eventually leads to the atrophy of the colon's muscles and nerves.

- Stress impairs digestion, creating nervous system responses that inhibit reflexes that facilitate bowel movements.
- Low stomach acid interrupts digestion and allows blocks of food to linger in the intestines.
- Lack of fiber inhibits colonic contractions.
- Food intolerances to items like gluten and dairy products irritate the intestines and interfere with colon function.

For the sake of your overall health, I will always urge you to try to get more exercise (at least a twenty- to thirty-minute walk a day), reduce your stress, stop smoking, make every effort to avoid secondhand smoke, and decrease your coffee intake to one cup daily max. In addition, the last three items on this list—low stomach acid, lack of fiber, and food intolerances—are specifically addressed by the Gut Flush Plan. By following the regimen, you will be able to wean yourself off coffee and laxatives and allow your body to void wastes without pain or strain, just as Mother Nature intended.

> *[Constipation is] the primary cause of nearly every disturbance of the human system.*
>
> —Renowned health practitioner NORMAN WALKER, who believed that 80 percent of all disease begins in the colon

Diarrhea

Chronic or intermittent diarrhea that does not resolve on its own after three days is another sign that your colon is suffering from Gut Grief. Some individuals develop diarrhea after the removal of the gallbladder or stomach surgery; in either of these situations, diarrhea may be normal and nothing to become overly concerned about unless it doesn't go away on its own in a reasonable time (do check with your doctor on this).

The causes of diarrhea are many: yeast overgrowth; bacterial, viral, or parasitic infections; food intolerances; irritable bowel syndrome; lack of enzymes; celiac disease; and medications like antibiotics, blood pressure meds, and antacids containing magnesium—a formidable albeit "natural" laxative. Thankfully, the protocols in the Gut Flush Plan are designed to eliminate and balance all of the underlying factors that are creating the diarrhea in the first place.

One particular type of bacteria, an anaerobic gram-positive rod known as C. difficile, considered the newest Superbug, is the most frequently identified cause of antibiotic-associated diarrhea (AAC). Many experts view this infection as more deadly than the MRSAs. It accounts for up to 25 percent of all episodes of AAC and is spreading in day-care centers, as well as becoming another epidemic in hospitals and long-term care facilities. Pathogenic strains of C. difficile produce two distinct toxins that cause serious mucosal inflammation and damage. Statistics show that when patients use conventional measures, 20 percent are prone to relapse and this little bugger gets harder and harder to eradicate with each relapse. The good news is that most patients improve with the very same probiotics treatment that Marty Jean used.

One caution: newborns and infants are most at risk if there is continuing severe diarrhea. Even a day or two can result in dehydration, so lots of liquids and electrolytes are in order. Of course, if the child is running a fever of 102 degrees, is complaining of severe abdominal pain, and their stools look bloody and tarry, call the doctor right away. Avoid milk products and fatty and sweet foods, and use the old-fashioned standby BRAT diet of bananas, rice, applesauce, and toast—usually it works quite well.

Interestingly, emotions can also play a role in recurring diarrhea. You have to keep in mind that, in a way, your gut has a brain of its very own and is very sensitive to stress. In fact, a whopping 95 percent of the body's serotonin (the brain's feel-good neurotransmitter) is located in the bowel. Serotonin is also needed for a smooth-functioning and healthy colon, as well as your brain. If stress and anxiety deplete this vital neurotransmitter, the bowel will also suffer. In fact, anger, hostility, and trauma can create malfunction in the form of diarrhea, so dealing with your emotions and seeing a professional counselor who specializes in emotional eating may be a major part of your entire recovery process (see Resources).

Diverticulosis

An increasingly common diagnosis these days is diverticulosis—it's become so prevalent that by the age of eighty-five a whopping two thirds of all Americans have it. It is thought to be caused by a lack of the right kind of fiber which creates a great deal of pressure on the outer muscles of the colon, resulting in a smaller and harder stool as well as major abdominal pain, cramps, gas, and bloating. A little sac called a diverticulum is formed as the colon bulges in certain places due to the increased pressure which makes the muscle fibers separate.

If the condition becomes diverticulitis, this advanced situation can become life-threatening. Food becomes trapped in the little sacs and starts an inflammatory process, which can create rupture and peritonitis, a huge risk factor for colon cancer.

The Gut Flush Plan emphasizes the importance of ingesting insoluble fiber on a daily basis to bulk up the stool so that the muscles in your colon don't have to strain so much to push it through. As we'll discuss in Chapter 7, "Step 1: Fortify," the first step of the plan also promotes the importance of drinking at least half of your body weight in ounces of water to help the fiber move through the system. In turn, both of these healing solutions help to alleviate the pressure that pooches out the diverticulum.

Heartburn, Acid Indigestion, and GERD

When it comes to digestion, you'd think food would move in only one direction: down. Right? But in the case of heartburn, acid indigestion, and gastroesophageal reflux disease (GERD), the typical American Food Fright diet can turn digestion upside down.

During the normal digestive process, food moves from the mouth down into the stomach during the first stage of its journey through the GI tract. The valve that sits at the bottom of your esophagus and the top of your stomach, the lower esophageal sphincter (LES), is supposed to be a one-way passage—food passes through the valve, into the stomach, the valve closes, and nothing is supposed to come back up.

Usually this process works just fine. The stomach receives food and secretes hydrochloric acid (HCl) to break down individual nutrients and kill most of the pathogens in the food. (Luckily, the stomach has that coating of mucus, which prevents the acid from eating through the stomach wall.) But when you consume too much coffee, chocolate, pepper, mints, alcohol,

COULD GERD BE JUST ANOTHER NAME FOR HIATAL HERNIA?

Gastroesophageal reflux disease, or GERD, may also be linked with a painful condition known as hiatal hernia. In fact, most individuals who suffer from acid reflux have a hiatal hernia. Coincidence? I think not. The literature suggests that more than 90 percent of those with acid reflux have a hiatal hernia, and when the hiatal hernia resolves, so does the acid reflux. It appears that both overweight and extreme flatulence are huge factors.

A hiatal hernia occurs when the upper part of the stomach pushes into the opening of the diaphragm and becomes stuck. Pain in the chest and back can intensify when intestinal gas pressures the stomach up into the esophagus, as it did in my own case. The resulting crowding of the stomach, heart, lungs, and nerves can make some sufferers feel like they have heart problems in addition to breathlessness, extreme bloating, and severe indigestion.

If you have acid reflux, it certainly wouldn't hurt to be checked out for a hiatal hernia. A naturopath or well-trained chiropractor may be able to perform some targeted soft-tissue manipulation to pull the hiatal hernia down where it belongs. For immediate relief, try this: drink two full glasses of warm water to help weigh your stomach down. After drinking the water, take a breath, jump slightly, and breathe out forcefully as you return to the floor. That allows gravity to pull your stomach (now filled with water) down as your diaphragm comes up. A mini-trampoline works well for this exercise.

onions, or processed foods with refined sugar, or a diet high in fat, you weaken the LES. The LES then fails to close properly, and the mix of HCl and undigested food flows back from the stomach into the esophagus, searing its sensitive tissues. That's when you feel the burning ring of fire of GERD, also known as acid reflux.

GERD is torture for many. About 21 million Americans suffer from some form of the disease, such as nausea, vomiting, or heartburn. These symptoms can be accompanied by bloating, gas, belching, rectal itches, and draining fatigue.

Alarmingly, the acid-suppressing drugs that are recommended for this condition (think Nexium and Prilosec) have recently been connected to a number of potentially dangerous side effects. These little-known but nasty side effects of the acid suppressors (also known as proton pump inhibitors, or PPIs) include an increased risk of pneumonia, infection with the Superbug C. difficile, and hip fractures because of osteoporosis. In 2006, the *Journal of the American Medical Association* reported an increased risk of hip fracture by 44 percent with patients taking the PPI drugs.

Happily, the Gut Flush Plan has some simple and safe solutions that will help you to deal with GERD. Hydrochloric acid is one of them. Jonathan Wright, M.D., a nutritional pioneer who is also an expert on hydrochloric acid, has found that some 90 percent of his patients who suffer from acid reflux have too little rather than too much HCl. His clinic in Tacoma, Washington, performs the Heidelberg test in which you swallow a small plastic capsule containing electronic monitoring equipment that can access your HCl levels (see Resources).

Ulcers

Many people think that if you worry a lot, you'll give yourself an ulcer. I can't tell you how many people with whom I consult still believe this myth. They think too much stress at work or at home, always being on the go, and never relaxing causes your stomach to make too much acid and, voilà, a stomach ulcer. If only it was that simple.

Yes, stress can contribute to or exacerbate an existing ulcer. But stress alone doesn't create one. Our Food Fright environment has contributed to ulcers and made them a serious problem that, along with the other symptoms of Gut Grief, is on the increase. About 70 percent of stomach ulcers have been linked to a specific Superbug bacteria, Heliobacter pylori, or H. pylori. Research shows that about half of the humans on Earth have H. pylori in their digestive tract. But not everyone develops ulcers; only when this bacteria grows out of control in the stomach or upper part of the small intestine does it lead to sores on the lining of the digestive tract.

Sufferers say ulcers feel like fire in the pit of your stomach, just under the breastbone, that worsens on an empty stomach. Ulcers can drain your energy, bleed, and cause your bowel movements to turn black. Some people don't feel any discomfort until the problem becomes serious; for others, ulcers are a painful recurring malady. A million Americans a year head to the hospital for ulcers, and about six thousand even lose their lives. As a result, the health care price for ulcers has now topped $6 billion every year.

Luckily, you can experience relief—and the Gut Flush Plan can help you avoid and even treat ulcers naturally with the right kind of probiotics and a resinlike supplement derived from the sap of pistachio trees targeted to neutralize H. pylori. And there is a simple, inexpensive "hot" culinary trick that will not only spice up your health but also inhibit the growth of H. pylori—even with the drug-resistant strains.

We've seen how the symptoms of Gut Grief can be uncomfortable, painful, even downright deadly. Now let's talk about solutions.

Mother Nature has built in all the necessary protections—we just need to learn how to properly maintain them in our Food Fright environment. The Gut Flush Plan reinforces the three most powerful natural defenses already present in your body—probiotics, hydrochloric acid, and digestive enzymes—so they can help restore your balance and ban Gut Grief for good.

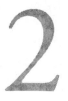

The GI's Good Guys: HCl, Probiotics, and Digestive Enzymes

WHEN MY CLIENT AMELIA CAME TO SEE ME AS A LAST RESORT, SHE WAS really full of it—full of gas and uninterrupted burping—even twenty-four to thirty-six hours after eating. She also suffered from bloating, anemia, the beginning stages of osteoporosis, and pressure around her heart. But what was most evident to me during my sessions with Amelia was her distraught mental state. She was always upset and very nervous.

After reviewing her blood tests and a two-week diet diary that revealed stellar food choices (lots of good protein, the right kind of essential fats, nongluten starches, assorted veggies, and moderate fruits), it finally dawned on me what was going on. No matter how good Amelia's diet was, her food was not being digested and her body not properly nourished because she was suffering from a deficiency of hydrochloric acid, suppressed by her emotions and constant worry. Upset emotions before or after a meal can halt the production of hydrochloric acid even if you normally have an adequate supply. So a top-notch diet with all the best protein in the world but without the hydrochloric acid won't do much good. And that goes for assimilating iron and calcium, too.

You'll hear me mention it many times throughout the book, so I want to make this very clear: a whole slew of diseases and uninvited "guests" have a much tougher time taking up residence in a healthy body than a weakened one.

For the most part, our body's natural defenses want to prevent us from catching germs and becoming host to every passing microbe or disease condition—we just have to do our part to support those defenses.

The main allies that fight on the side of smooth digestion and good health are our natural stomach acid, or hydrochloric acid (HCl); probiotics, the friendly bacteria that inhabit your entire digestive system; and digestive enzymes, catalysts that facilitate and speed the breakdown of food in the stomach. HCl, probiotics, and digestive enzymes all labor tirelessly in alliance with the colon and the immune system to make sure your gastrointestinal system stays on track and doesn't succumb to the yeast, pathogens, and other meddlers that can turn your gut into their nasty playground. Because of their power to right the wrongs of Gut Grief, HCl, probiotics, and digestive enzymes form the foundation of the Gut Flush Plan.

Let's look at HCl first.

Hydrochloric Acid, the *Good* Stomach Acid

For years we talked about "acid stomach" being a bad thing. People would drink milk or chug Pepto-Bismol to tame a burning belly, and everyone would blame the fire on too much stomach acid. But rather than needing to decrease the amount of acid in our stomach, we actually need to *increase* it. It turns out that HCl is a potent sterilizer of all kinds of contaminates, due to its highly acidic pH. Outside your body, HCl is actually strong enough to burn a hole in your carpet!

HCl is your body's front line of defense against hostile gas-producing bacteria and parasites, so low levels of HCl make us more susceptible to infections from Salmonella and other bugs in food and water. In addition, a lowered level of HCl leads to malabsorption, poor assimilation, and ineffective distribution of essential nutrients, such as sodium, iron, calcium, and magnesium. Fifteen minerals, eight essential amino acids, and numerous vitamins depend on HCl for absorption. For example, no matter how much calcium you take in supplement form, if your stomach acid drops too low, those supplements won't help you prevent osteoporosis. Similarly, supplements with iron won't help strengthen your blood without stomach acid to help you absorb this crucial mineral. Lowered levels of HCl can also lead to an underfunctioning liver and pancreas, a deficit of potassium (essential for the heart), and the formation of boils, abscesses, and puss. Not good!

Sadly, because of several factors in our Food Fright environment, our levels of HCl may be declining at the very moment when we need HCl most. Medical professionals have long believed that stomach acid production declines by half after you reach age forty. But based on the work I've done with thousands of people, I think we need to revise that thinking. A lack of stomach acid has become much more widespread, and these days, almost everyone, at every age, suffers from this condition.

One overriding factor in our national HCl shortage is stress. We are all gulping down our food, eating much too quickly, eating irregularly, drinking large amounts of fluids with meals, swallowing air when we're eating, and crowding in way too much food at one time. These kinds of stressors conspire to slow down our secretion of stomach acid. The popularity of low-carbohydrate diets has also made the stomach acid problem much worse. That's because the large amount of protein in such a diet overwhelms your HCl production. Your body can't produce enough HCl to break down the protein. Consequently, you end up with undigested food, indigestion, and constipation.

In addition, if you drink too much water, especially cold water, while you eat or within two hours of eating, you disrupt your stomach acid function. Or if you don't chew your food enough. Or if your diet lacks A and B vitamins or zinc or iodine or salt. Or if you have medical X-rays, drink chlorinated water . . . the list goes on and on. Dozens of factors in our Food Fright environment steal your valuable stomach acid and can leave you with gas, bloating, acid reflux, heartburn, constipation, and diarrhea—and sometimes even worse.

Is your HCl low? If you're curious about the level of HCl in your system, you can try the self-test (see "HCl Stomach Acid Test," page 19). In the meantime, consider these signs that you might have too little HCl:

- a sense of feeling full almost as soon as you start eating
- belching and bloating

- gassiness
- nausea and vomiting
- losing your taste for meat
- heartburn and burning in your stomach
- sour taste in your mouth
- bad breath
- chronic yeast infections
- weak nails
- rectal itching
- hoarseness and laryngitis
- rosacea

Following the Gut Flush Plan is a big step toward buttressing your lagging HCl production and helping ban Gut Grief. To kick off the program, and to help your system get the HCl it desperately needs, I will recommend HCl supplements as part of the basic protocol for the Gut Flush Plan (see "The Gut Flush Basic Protocol," page 26). But before we get to that, let's

---

A SHORTAGE OF HCL

While many if not most of us suffer from a lack of stomach acid, certain people are more susceptible to declining HCl. Your stomach acid may be low if you've been told you have:

- gastroesophageal reflux disorder (GERD)
- deficiency in protein, calcium, magnesium, and/or iron
- immune disorders
- arthritis
- hives
- osteoporosis
- hepatitis
- gallbladder disease
- lupus
- vitiligo

To check to see if you have adequate stomach acid, try this home test. (Do not do this test if you have ulcers or a preulcerative condition.)

- Take an HCl (betaine hydrochloride) supplement of 500–550 milligrams and 150 milligrams of pepsin with your next meal. (Note: HCl should not be taken simultaneously with anti-inflammatory medications like Indocin, Butazolidin, aspirin, or Motrin.) If you have trouble finding an HCl supplement that meets the dosage criteria, do consider HCl+2, the supplement I created for my own clients. (It also contains bile acids for healthy fat digestion, so you get a double whammy of digestive help.) (See Resoures.)

- Observe how you feel. Extreme warmth signals that you have sufficient stomach acid and means you should discontinue the supplements or cut back.

- If you experience no relief from your digestive problems, or feel no pain or warmth, double your HCl dose at the next meal.

- Continue adding an extra dose per meal until you feel warmth. Caution: Don't take more than five tablets at a time.

- At succeeding meals after you reach your limit, take one less than your maximum with food.

- After three to six months try reducing your dosage.

learn about Mother Nature's second, and perhaps greatest, ally for you in the fight against Gut Grief: probiotics.

Probiotics, the *Good* Bacteria

Quick: Where is your immune system? If you're not sure, you're not alone. Most people have no idea where the immune system resides in the body—they're apt to think of it almost as a mythical force field. In reality, 60 percent of your immune system's receptor cells are in your colon and another 15 percent are in the lower part of the small intestine. That means 75 percent of your body's immune system is at the mercy of the goings-on in your gut.

In a healthy colon, an almost countless number of friendly bacteria, or probiotics, help these immune system receptor cells do their defensive job. Probiotics inhabit the walls of the small intestine and the colon, fortifying them, forming a protective barrier that makes it harder for pathogenic bugs like E. coli and Salmonella to take root and multiply.

Ideally, beneficial probiotic bacteria make up about 85 percent of bacteria in your GI tract. To date, scientists have identified about one hundred different kinds of probiotic bacteria. Of these, Lactobacillus acidophilus, commonly found in yogurt, is probably the best known. Most prevalent in the small intestine where it partners with the immune system, Lactobacillus acidophilus helps digest proteins, carbs, and milk sugar and produces the lactic acid compounds that make the digestive tract acidic enough to deter potentially dangerous bacteria. Another well-known bacterial family, the bifidobacteria, primarily populates the large intestine, where they ferment soluble fiber to feed the colon's cells and keep pathogens at bay.

As long as these beneficial bacteria dominate, and hover around this 85 percent mark, the other 15 percent of harmful bacteria usually don't present a problem. In a healthy gut, probiotic cells would number around 100 billion to 1,000 billion per milliliter of digestive tract. This number ensures that probiotics have a majority strong enough to do their best job protecting your health. But when the balance starts to tip, "bad" bacteria overgrow and can cause serious health risks. Today, many Americans have friendly flora counts as low as 5 per milliliter. Not 5 billion—just *five*. That's not just a drop—that's a probiotic meltdown.

As the probiotics dwindle in the colon, so does your health. When the good bacteria disappear, bad ones rush in to take their place on the walls of the colon. Once that happens, all sorts of pathogens can gain a foothold in your gut and spread their toxins into the entire body. The colon (and the rest of the body) can be overrun by detrimental microorganisms like virulent Salmonella, E. coli, H. pylori (the ulcer-causing bacteria we spoke of earlier), C. difficile (antibiotic-associated diarrhea), and the notorious antibiotic-resistant MRSA staph infections that have been a menace in hospitals for years and that are now spreading into the community.

Many surprising conditions, such as asthma, sinusitis, and kidney stones, can be traced back to imbalances of the beneficial and harmful bacteria in your GI tract. E. coli, for example, can disrupt the way insulin controls your blood sugar and make you more vulnerable to diabetes. The lack of beneficial bacteria and the expansion of Superbugs can also lead to the accumulation of endotoxins, biologically active substances that can cause great damage in the body. In hospitals, experts estimate, about fifty thousand people die every year from endotoxin-induced shock. In the gastrointestinal tract, the presence of endotoxins can exacerbate pancreatitis while leading to skin problems like psoriasis or autoimmune disorders like lupus erythematosus.

Since the good bacteria normally partner with immune cells to keep out the Superbugs and pathogens, dwindling numbers of beneficial bacteria can trigger your immune system to become consistently overstimulated. This results in localized inflammation, which then produces a rippling effect throughout the entire body. Inflammation can severely aggravate arthritis and set off rheumatic health issues; it can lead to cramps, diarrhea, even high blood pressure and heart disease.

To make matters worse, as you run short of probiotics, your digestion is impeded, allowing partially broken down protein fragments to be absorbed into the bloodstream. Their presence there, where they don't belong, can further aggravate nervous system problems, increase eczema, and increase your susceptibility to a variety of allergies. Loss of probiotics can even lead to a failure of the recirculation of female hormones such as estrogen.

And all this medical heartache basically results from the simple turf war between two bacterial factions.

How did we get here, you ask? Just how have we allowed this probiotic meltdown to happen? It comes down to two critical missteps:

- As a nation, we are unknowingly eating more nationally distributed foods—foods that are making Food Fright headlines and that not only starve our natural probiotics but actively kill them; and perhaps most important,
- As a nation, we've become completely addicted to the casual, thoughtless use of antibiotics.

For years Americans have ignored the warnings of scientists who urged us to curb our unnecessary use of antibiotics everywhere from our food supply to our medicine cabinets. As a result, we've been coconspirators in a wide-spread extermination of the very flora that protect our health. Our casual addiction to antibiotics, when combined with several other Food Fright factors, has simultaneously crippled probiotics and emboldened pathogenic bugs, enabling them to strengthen and multiply to such a degree that they now threaten our lives. Let's look more closely at these probiotic killers.

The antibiotics in our food supply kill probiotics. Along with bacteria-tainted food, we routinely swallow low levels of secondhand antibiotics contained in commercial meat and dairy products. These secondhand antibiotics, like any antibiotic, can deplete all bacteria in your intestines, including the friendly bacteria.

Fifty million pounds of antibiotics are used each year in the United States and up to 18 million pounds are routinely placed in food and water of even healthy livestock. They're used in fisheries and on poultry. Farmers use them so they can raise more animals in closer quarters without disease wiping out the whole herd. Cows are given antibiotics because they make them grow bigger, increasing the farmer's return on investment.

And, inevitably, these antibiotics end up on the end of our forks.

The meats we broil, the chicken we grill, and the fish we steam often contain low levels of antibiotic residues—no matter how healthy the cooking methods. Those low levels of antibiotics are the most destructive—just strong enough to allow pathogens in your body to develop resistance to these drugs but not strong enough to totally wipe them out.

The antibiotics in our medicine chests kill probiotics. While pharmaceutical antibiotics are certainly helpful against bacterial infection, we've been using way too many of them for our own good. Experts estimate that doctors hand out 20 million prescriptions a year for unnecessary antibiotics when the real cause is a virus like the common cold, which can't be "cured" by antibiotics. Research shows that common maladies like young children's ear infections are often better left to run their course even though many pediatricians prescribe antibiotics. Another study in the *New England Journal of Medicine* found that antibiotics are being unnecessarily prescribed for conditions like acute bronchitis, which, like the common cold, are often caused by a virus. Dr. David Bell, assistant director of the National Center for Infectious Diseases (part of the Centers for Disease Control), is not crying wolf when he says, "Virtually every important human infection is becoming resistant to the drug of choice used to treat it in the United States and all over the world."

Why do doctors keep prescribing antibiotics unnecessarily, despite years of warnings from the CDC and other influential medical organizations? Why do consumers keep buying antibacterial products that do little other than breed Superbugs? I think this denial is, in part, human nature—we have a "not in my backyard" fear reflex that seeks to protect our personal safety as it denies our personal responsibility. Because we are terrified of the alternatives—bacterial infections picked up at random—we all tend to feel that antibiotic resistance is someone else's problem. We want to keep ourselves and our families safe from bugs, so we don't think about the long-term, societal ramifications of that "just in case" antibiotic prescription or antibacterial hand soap. We need to start thinking about the bigger picture—and the responsible food and lifestyle choices on the Gut Flush Plan not only help protect you and your family, it can help protect the environment as well.

PROBIOTICS: KILLED BY FRIENDLY FIRE

When you look at the way our lifestyles and diets do so little to support the probiotics in our gut, maybe it's a miracle that any of the friendly bacteria in our digestive tract have survived at all up to this point. With friends like us, probiotics don't need enemies like E. coli, Candida, and Salmonella.

You're destroying probiotics if you:

- take antibiotics for viral diseases like the common cold; the cold virus isn't touched by antibiotics but these medications wipe out probiotics;
- eat nonorganic meat, which often contains antibiotic residues;
- overuse antiseptic natural agents like oregano oil, echinacea, barberry, colloidal silver, and goldenseal;
- drink chlorinated and fluoridated water;
- lead an overstressed lifestyle;
- Eat processed and sugary foods, which encourage the growth of pathogenic bacteria in our intestinal tract. The more refined sugar you eat, the more probiotics you need.

Other Food Fright choices kill probiotics. Antibiotics are probably the most potent robbers of beneficial bacteria, but other elements also alter the optimal balance of these beneficial bacteria—or even destroy it outright. These seemingly unrelated factors include: sugar, alcohol, stress, oral contraceptives and steroids, drugs, chlorinated drinking water, X-ray/radiation exposure, and even natural health food antiseptic aids like oil of oregano and colloidal silver.

In addition, as a culture, we've stopped eating fermented foods like sauerkraut, kimchi (the Korean version of sauerkraut), kefir, and tempeh that in past epochs were a crucial part of the human diet. These foods, which have been given short shrift in the supermarket, "feed" and sustain the probiotic population in our digestive tracts. We've also omitted fiber from our diet, but fiber is a key nutrient that helps intestinal probiotics thrive. All the while, we've indulged in the sugary and refined foods that are manna to pathogens: yeast, infectious bacteria, and parasites thrive on a diet filled with sweets. The Gut Flush Plan rights these nutritional imbalances and puts more probiotic and "prebiotic" foods back where they belong, front and center of the dinner plate. (We'll talk more about these beneficial foods in chapters 3 and 5, as well as throughout *The Gut Flush Plan*.)

In a frightening way, our modern lifestyle has made it nearly impossible for beneficial bacteria to thrive. As the MRSA epidemic has shown us, we are now at a crisis point. Without a proper supply of these probiotics, the colon is practically defenseless against attack—valuable nutrients go unabsorbed, immune functions are impeded, pathogens accumulate, and the dangerous bacteria in our food find it easier to infect us. As a result, we will suffer increasing tides of allergies, irritable bowel syndrome, ulcerative colitis, asthma, yeast infections—and these are just the beginning. That's why the basic Gut Flush protocol includes a daily supplement of probiotics (see "The Gut Flush Basic Protocol," page 26).

Depleted beneficial bacteria combined with a lack of hydrochloric acid usually leads to a deficiency in other digestive enzymes as well. The lack of all of these protective elements (probiotics, HCl, and digestive enzymes) prevent you from digesting, absorbing, and assimilating your food, creating an onslaught of problems for your body. Let's consider the third ally in Mother Nature's arsenal against Gut Grief: digestive enzymes.

Digestive Enzymes

You've probably heard a lot about enzymes but, like many people, have no idea what they do or how they do it. While their role is controversial, most experts would agree that digestive enzymes are catalysts that speed the breakdown of food into its elemental parts—carbohydrates, protein, and fat—so it can be absorbed through the walls of the digestive tract. Our bodies produce three main categories of enzymes: amylases that break down carbs, proteases that cleave proteins, and lipases that decompose fats.

Enzymes begin interacting with food as soon as we start to chew. The amylases in saliva begin to tear apart starch into sugars. As you swallow your chewed food, the stomach sends out hormones to the pancreas and gallbladder that stimulate them to make enzymes to further break down your meal. (The pancreas releases upward of 1.5 liters of digestive juices into the small intestine every day!) If you've had some protein in your meal, protease enzymes help liberate the protein's amino acids so they can take on a form more readily absorbed into the bloodstream.

Once your food is broken down into smaller nutrients, various sections of the small intestine use a complex set of chemical processes to pick and choose what to absorb and release into the circulatory system. If anything goes wrong with this process, you experience the flatulence, bloating, and indigestion that can make you feel miserable. Partially digested foods can create toxins as they travel through your system, resulting in food allergies and the overgrowth of pathogenic bacteria, which can then produce endotoxins and other byproducts that overload your GI tract. So you can see that enzymes are very critical to digestive health.

Natural health practitioners believe that eating raw foods, like fresh fruits and vegetables, which are rich in enzymes, can help our bodies supply sufficient enzymes to better digest our food. Many so-called "traditional" societies ate much greater quantities of these types of raw foods, including raw meats, raw fish, and raw dairy products. Raw food advocates argue that our Food Fright diet, heavily laden with cooked and processed foods, is missing out on enzymes, forcing our pancreases to work much harder to produce enzymes for digestion. This need for enhanced enzyme production can compromise our health by putting extra burdens on the pancreas.

These days, of course, many raw foods may be too contaminated with dangerous pathogens to consume safely. That's why I recommend enzyme supplementation as well as the addition of fermented foods that have extra enzymes created by the probiotics in these dishes.

Although research has not precisely identified why, stress also seems to be one of the most important influences on how our bodies produce enzymes. Scientists have found that stress significantly changes the enzymes found in saliva to such a degree that they now use the measurement of enzymes as a gauge of people's stress levels.

If you are under a lot of stress and experiencing bloating, flatulence, and indigestion, you are probably lacking digestive enzymes, as well as hydrochloric acid and probiotics. Along with stress and a poor diet, advancing age and an unhealthy environment can all contribute to a decrease in your digestive enzyme production. To help remedy this all-too-common situation, I recommend a broad-based enzyme as part of the Gut Flush Basic Protocol to support digestive enzyme activity in the body.

The Gut Flush Basic Protocol

Now that you know about Mother Nature's three miracle helpers, you're ready to begin the Gut Flush Plan. We'll start with the Gut Flush Basic Protocol, a daily regimen that will help everyone, no matter what your particular brand of Gut Grief.

The three main objectives of the Gut Flush Plan are:

- to increase the number of probiotics;
- to increase the level of HCl;
- to increase the activity of digestive enzymes in our system.

Every suggestion, every food or lifestyle change I'll recommend will, in some way, impact or enhance these three allies of the digestive tract.

HCl, probiotics, and digestive enzymes are all critical to smooth digestive functioning, and each already exists in the body. Almost everyone can feel confident beginning with this protocol; the only caution I would make is for those already taking certain medications under a doctor's care or who have an ulcer (please check with your doctor first).

For best results, follow the specific advice about dosage and timing. These supplements are available online at UniKeyHealth.com or similar formulations can be found at most health food stores throughout the country.

1. **Probiotics:** When you first begin the program, take a loading dose of Dr. Ohhira's Probiotics 12 PLUS: Five capsules in the a.m. on an empty stomach; five capsules in the p.m. on an empty stomach. After five days, switch to the maintenance dose of two capsules in the a.m. on an empty stomach and two in the p.m. on an empty stomach.
2. **HCl:** Take two or more HCl + 2 (hydrocholric acid with pepsin and bile salts for added fat digestion) with meals.
3. **Digestive enzymes:** Daily with meals take 1 to 3 tablets derived from pancreatin or papaya. I prefer American Biologics Ultra Infl-Zyme, which contains pancreatin, bromelain, papain, chymotrypsin, trypsin, and lipase as well as other helpful ingredients. This product can be used as a digestive aid with meals or as a natural anti-inflammatory between meals at the same dosage.

Once you've taken the Gut Flush Basic Protocol for a few days, you should notice a dramatic increase in energy, better regularity, and calmer nerves. If you experience more gas, don't worry: the friendly flora are going to war against your internal pathogens, which is a good thing, a very good thing indeed. Sometimes it takes two weeks or sometimes two months for the gut to settle down—but no matter how long, you will be insured for enhanced immunity and quality longer.

As you progress on the Gut Flush Plan, add in any protocols specific to your situation, and then enjoy the three-week meal plan; you'll notice you will gradually experience less constipation, diarrhea, gas, bloating, lack of energy, acid reflux and poor concentration, and fewer persistent aches and pains, yeast infections, and even emotional problems. Now, granted—it's not going to happen overnight; gut flushing is an evolving lifestyle process designed to change the way you approach your daily habits, diet, and food safety practices that can seriously undermine your well-being. But with the Gut Flush Basic Protocol, no matter what your condition, you can start making headway today.

Now that you're off on your running start, let's take a moment to consider your specific situation. Many of us, myself included, go for months or even years suffering from Gut Grief without any idea of where it comes from. The frightening truth is that the vast majority of us are unknowing hosts or victims of what I call the Colon Corruptors: yeast, parasites, Superbugs, and food sensitivities. Before you can get the maximum benefit out of the Gut Flush Plan to Fortify, Flush, and Feed your digestive system, you need to recognize the symptoms of any individual pathogens or sensitivities that may be lurking behind the scenes.

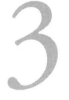

Colon Corruptor #1: Yeast

I REMEMBER SOMEBODY ONCE SAYING THAT IT TAKES A YEAR FOR YOUR system to recover from a single course of antibiotics. In my case, it took a year and a half.

By the time I was fifty, it had literally been decades since I had taken an antibiotic, for anything. As a teenager, I took tetracycline for my skin—that might have been the last time. That is, until my left eyelid started to act up at the age of fifty-plus and I developed not one but several sties. (In retrospect, I see that these eye maladies usually occur when I am not "seeing" things clearly, and that was definitely the case when my lid started to act up—but that's another story.)

Since I have always taken probiotics and used HCl as well as digestive enzymes, I figured that if anybody's system could withstand a ten-day course of antibiotics, my system certainly could. The first sty blossomed right before a trip back East during which I was scheduled to make several guest appearances. My eye doctor believed that the sties would go away faster if I was "proactive" with the antibiotics. Well, perhaps you already know the end to this story—suffice it to say, they didn't.

All told, it took a full two months for the sties to clear up. In the interim, I decided it was also time to do some remedial dental work for cavitations, a process that reams out small holes in the bones where a tooth has been pulled and where bacteria gather and then seep into the system. Enlightened dentists, like the renowned Hal Huggins, DDS, M.S., believe that the endotoxins from these bone-infecting bacteria are more toxic than botulism and can infect any system of the body: the heart, the brain, the gut, the breast, the lungs—whichever is your "weakest link." So, no wonder my stool analysis uncovered such virulent and inflammatory bacteria. In my case, tooth Number 29 was the problem area, and this particular tooth (based upon energetic medicine and the acupuncture meridian zones) was related to my stomach, pyloric valve, sinuses, and pancreas; no matter what I was doing, the constant bacterial poisoning of my system coupled with the antibiotics was wreaking havoc on my digestion. Since the local dentist who performed the cavitation wanted to err on the side of caution, I was prescribed still another dose of antiobiotics.

It gets worse from here. As you know, stress can be draining on so many levels. So when this ongoing antibiotic therapy was added to some inordinate stress brought on by a deeply disturbing business deal gone bad, the results were disastrous.

The antibiotics caused major yeast overgrowth which in turn pushed up my stomach to create a hiatal hernia. The pain was so great that I thought I was having a heart attack. I realize now that I should have been shoring up my probiotics and the rest of my nutrients triplefold. While I had continued to take the Gut Flush Basic Protocol, I should have gone back to the "loading" dose. I neglected to do so because, well, I am human and didn't take the time to really take care of myself. And, ultimately, that oversight cost me dearly.

You would think I, of all people, should have known better. But when you are in the midst of pain and not knowing what is really wrong with you, anxiety sets in and you can't be objective, especially with yourself.

Finally, I was able to resolve the source of my most puzzling gut discomforts with the help of a biofeedback machine that kept registering "dental" on its evaluation scan. A year later I was reevaluated for the cavitation and learned via panoramic X-ray and a special ultrasound scan on my mouth that the hole in my jawbone hadn't healed. I then contacted Hal Huggins, who put me in touch with one of his dental associates who had overcome Lou Gehrig's disease by removing toxic dental materials and cleaning up root canals and cavitations. (See Resources.) Now my story has a happy ending. After a full year of doubt, worry, concern, and frustration (I did every diagnostic test known to Western medicine, just in case), my gut is back to its happy self. And yours can be, too—that's my promise to you.

For your sake, I hope you've not experienced anything quite as troubling or painful as what I endured. But if you have, you owe it to yourself to find out why. Until you get to the bottom of your particular gastrointestinal upset, you may never get the full benefit of the Gut Flush Plan.

Throughout the years that I've been working with clients I've discovered that most digestive woes can be traced back to four specific sources: yeast, parasites, Superbugs, or food sensitivities. In the next four chapters, we'll consider each of these in turn. At the end of each chapter, you'll find a brief self-test that can help you determine if your own symptoms have their origins with one of the Colon Corruptors. (In order to get a definitive diagnosis, you may have to consult a doctor or a testing lab.) You'll also find a specific protocol that will help you treat your condition or prevent that particular foe from gaining traction again. Since it's one of the most common infestations, let's look at yeast first.

The Fungus Among Us

You just can't escape yeast. Candida albicans is in the air, in your throat, and in your gut. That's a fact of life. This yeast is everywhere, coexisting with all the other microorganisms that fill the microscopic spaces of the world. But when Candida grows out of control you can end up with many seemingly disconnected symptoms, including intense fatigue, sinus pain, headaches, joint problems, and urinary infections.

You can't totally eliminate Candida, but normally your probiotic defenses work with your immune system to keep these potential troublemakers in the minority. As the natural balance of microorganisms in our bodies breaks down, however—under pressure from Food Fright, pollutants, toxins, and the overall stress of everyday life—one in three adults, mostly women, experience the discomforts of candidiasis overgrowth. That's about 90 million of us on any given day. In my mind, that easily qualifies as another epidemic.

Yeast is like a super villain with a secret identity. When yeast cells are under control, these single, mild-mannered elliptical cells reside on the mucous membranes of the gastrointestinal tract and peacefully coexist with the other denizens of the intestines.

But give them a chance to multiply and take a majority position, and their mild manners fade and they quickly overwhelm the body's defensive mechanisms. In this attack mode, single cells of Candida join and work in unison to form long threads called hyphae. These rootlike structures drill into the walls of the intestines and also bore into macrophages, the immune cells that normally kill Candida. This process funnels fungus, toxins, and other debris (such as undigested fragments of protein) directly into blood vessels and other organs.

As yeast spreads, reproduces, and distributes its toxic entourage, almost any part of your body may suffer symptoms. You may feel:

- intense fatigue, headaches, insomnia, weight fluctuations (up and down), mood swings, pain, jittery feelings, appetite loss, agitation;
- bloating, flatulence, indigestion, constipation, diarrhea, stomach pain, stools filled with mucus;
- burning, frequent, and/or urgent urination, recurring bladder infections, cystitis;
- cramps, irregular periods, depression, severe PMS symptoms;
- itching, burning, white vaginal discharge;
- dry mouth, rashes, sore and/or bleeding gums, white patches;
- nasal itching and sinus congestion;
- psoriasis, rashes, acne;
- burning sensations in the eyes, blurry vision, chronic inflammation, tearing, sudden changes in vision;
- loss of hearing, fluid in inner ear, recurring infections, ear pain.

Yeast overgrowth is so prevalent, and its symptoms are so widespread, it's often hard to zero in on the causes. Luckily, we know several risk factors which greatly increase your chances of encouraging Candida overgrowth. Once you are aware of these, you can begin to minimize their impact on your health.

Risk Factors for Yeast Overgrowth

Many of our difficulties with yeast are the unintended consequences of lifestyle habits that were supposed to bring better health or help us lose weight. Let's consider some of the most common risk factors for yeast overgrowth.

Repeated antibiotics. Those repeated doses of antibiotics we discussed in Chapter 1, as well as birth control pills, afford yeast the chance to overgrow. Antibiotics kill off all bacteria, including the beneficial probiotics that would otherwise block yeast from adhering to the intestinal walls.

Compromised immunity. Anything that weakens your immune system offers yeast an enhanced prospect for furthering its own interests at your expense. Medications such as steroids and other pharmaceuticals that restrain the immune system often have side effects that include decreased resistance to yeast. And a study in the peer-reviewed journal *Infections in Medicine* showed that Candida infections all by themselves can sap the immune system's ability to defend against future infections.

Cool, rainy climates. Many of my clients with the toughest cases of candidiasis live in and around San Francisco. This cool, perpetually damp part of the West Coast has a climate that Candida seems to love. As a matter of fact, when my client Penelope, who had struggled with years of yeast problems, finally moved to the drier, desert climate of southern California, her candidiasis cleared up almost instantly.

Being female. Women are yeast's favorite victims, since their internal environment offers up the most tempting terrain for candidiasis:

- Frequent fluctuations of hormones in the female body (including menstrual periods, pregnancies, and birth control pills) decrease immune defenses against candidiasis.
- Women's short urethras make them more prone to urinary infections, a circumstance that also increases vulnerability to yeast. Urinary infections

lead to more frequent rounds of antibiotics which, in turn, kill off the beneficial bacteria that help keep yeast in check.

- The vagina, dark and moist, offers a custom-made environment for yeast growth.
- Teenage girls take frequent rounds of antibiotics to quell acne; those treatments make them more susceptible to yeast overgrowth.
- Adult women visit physicians more frequently and are more likely to receive antibiotics for various conditions like sore throats and chest colds; those rounds of antibiotics create even more opportunities for yeast.

Low-fat, high-carb/good-carb diets. As we all know by now, our misguided quest to cut the fat in our diets, and our resulting binge on carbohydrate-rich foods, did not help us drop pounds. Instead of losing weight, we've become way more vulnerable to yeast. Fungus needs food, and sweets and starches keep yeast happily well fed. Even if you eat whole grains, any meal with excess carbs is a feast for yeast. In fact, your body needs certain kinds of fat to fight yeast.

Research from Japan shows that oleic acid, a type of monounsaturated fatty acid, inhibits Candida's shift from harmless, scattered cells to evil invader. When eaten, these fatty acids become part of the structure of the body's cellular membranes, helping limit the permeability of organs and tissues and shoring up the mucous membrane. Yeast cannot penetrate the blood, so it stays within its normal boundaries, in the intestinal tract and vaginal area, where it is less able to cause trouble. Rich sources of oleic acid are oils such as olive and sesame, which are both included in the various stages of the 21-Day Gut Flush Plan. Also noteworthy are the medium chain fatty acids in coconut oil, which have potent antifungal properties and leave the good bacteria alone. Coconut oil is featured in Week Two of the plan. Perhaps the best fat for fighting yeast are the omega-3s, as they fit best into the cell's structural membrane and provide fortification from the get-go. In Chapter 7 you'll learn more about how omega-3s fortify the gut against the Colon Corruptors, but for now, I encourage you to partake of a tablespoon of omega-3 fish oil or flaxseed oil right from the start.

Nutrient deficiencies. When you lack certain key minerals or your body isn't using them efficiently, your internal defenses against yeast fall apart. For example, while copper is necessary for Candida control a deficiency can make you more vulnerable to yeast, but ironically many "copperheads" find themselves troubled by a simultaneous excess and shortage of copper. They have high levels of copper stored in their tissues, but the copper is in an unbound form and therefore not bioavailable (the body isn't able to access the copper and properly use it).

Where is the excess copper coming from? It is coming mainly from environmental and "internal" sources, such as copper water pipes, copper IUDs, and silver amalgam fillings after 1976. Even malfunctioning adrenal glands can impact copper storage and utilization.

While copper is a vital weapon that can kill Candida, an excess of bioavailable copper can also cause problems; it's been shown to increase the pathogenic nature of Candida. Too much copper can therefore cause yeast infections to spread and worsen in intensity.

Optimal copper levels in blood and tissues are essential for both preventing and controlling the overgrowth of yeast. Many of my clients who had persistent yeast infections that didn't respond well to medical treatment found that their yeast problems disappeared after they got rid of their copper overload.

Other nutrients, such as zinc and biotin, a member of the B vitamins, also shore up immune defenses; shortages of these key nutrients give Candida a greater chance to convert into more harmful forms.

Underactive thyroid. In addition, thyroid insufficiency also interferes with your yeast defenses. Experts say that one in ten Americans has a thyroid that's not operating at full steam. This figure rises to one in five of postmenopausal women. So have your thyroid tested, especially your TSH, for starters.

Do You Have Excess Yeast?

Yeast overgrowth has so many diverse symptoms that self-diagnosis is difficult and often incorrect. Tempting though it may be, you should not attempt to self-diagnose candidiasis. Still, because Candida is so ubiquitous, a standard lab test may not give you an unqualified answer about your status. The only dependable method for a firm diagnosis of this yeast problem is for you and your health care provider to go over your medical history and symptoms and see if therapy helps alleviate your problems.

While the following diagnostic survey doesn't provide a definitive answer about the presence of Candida overgrowth I have found it helpful in identifying Candida's potential role in several health problems in adults. The survey was originally put together by the late William Crook, M.D., a Jackson, Tennessee, allergist, lecturer, and author of several books, including *The Yeast Connection and Women's Health* and *The Yeast Connection Cookbook.*

Dr. Crook spent the major part of his medical career documenting and fighting yeast overgrowth. He was a wonderful personal friend and colleague of mine. Up until he died in his early eighties, he persistently pursued new data about this health issue, and his work is still being confirmed by new studies and medical research that links yeast to premenstrual syndrome (PMS), psoriasis, multiple sclerosis, endometriosis, autism, interstitial cystitis, asthma, and chronic fatigue.

If you experience any of these health problems, note the number of points for that question. When you finish the questionnaire, add up the total points. Your final score indicates the probability that your health problems are linked to yeast overgrowth.

1. Have you taken repeated or prolonged courses of antibiotics?   *4 points*
2. Have you been bothered by recurrent vaginal, prostate, or urinary infections?   *3 points*
3. Do you feel "sick all over," yet the cause has not been found?   *2 points*
4. Are you bothered by hormone disturbances, including PMS, menstrual irregularities, sexual dysfunction, sugar cravings, low body temperature, or fatigue?   *2 points*
5. Are you unusually sensitive to tobacco smoke, perfumes and colognes, and chemical odors?   *2 points*
6. Are you bothered by memory or concentration problems? Do you sometimes feel spaced out or in a brain fog?   *2 points*
7. Have you taken a prolonged course of prednisone or other steroids, or have you taken birth control pills for more than three years?   *2 points*

8. Do some foods disagree with you or trigger your symptoms? *1 point*

9. Do you suffer with constipation, diarrhea, bloating, or abdominal pain? *1 point*

10. Does your skin itch, tingle, or burn; or is it unusually dry; or are you bothered by rashes? *1 point*

Women's scores: If you score 9 or more, your health problems are probably linked to yeast overgrowth. If you score 12 or more, your health problems are almost certainly connected to yeast.

Men's scores: If you score 7 or more, your health problems are most likely linked to yeast. A score of 10 or more indicates that your health problems are almost certainly connected to yeast.

THE GUT FLUSH FOOD BATH

To make produce last longer and kill off bacteria, fungus, and parasites that are in foods, use the Clorox bath pioneered by my mentor, Dr. Hazel Parcells. My clients and I have been using this method for more than thirty years and have survived many Food Fright epidemics.

- Use 1 teaspoon of Clorox to 1 gallon of purified, ozonated, and/or electrolyte-enhanced water.
- Place the foods to be treated into the bath for the length of time designated in the accompanying chart.
- Remove the food from the Clorox bath; place it in clear water for 10 minutes and rinse.
- Dry all foods thoroughly and store.

Leafy vegetables	15 minutes
Root, thick-skinned, or fibrous vegetables	30 minutes
Thin-skinned fruits, including berries, plums, peaches, and apricots	30 minutes
Thick-skinned fruits, including citrus, bananas, and apples	30 minutes
Poultry, fish, meat, and eggs	20 minutes

The Gut Flush Anti-Yeast Protocol

Yeast is primarily a problem of good versus evil—if you fortify your defensive forces, yeast will never have a chance. If your results from the survey above indicate that you may have a problem with yeast, try these suggestions to help tip the balance in your favor. Note: In my experience, one firm set of guidelines doesn't fit all. You may have to tweak these suggestions to find exactly the right fit that benefits your body most effectively.

Eliminate yeast, mold and nonprobiotic fermented foods, beverages, and condiments: As a first line of defense, I recommend that you use the Gut Flush Food Bath to help you kill any yeast that might be lingering on your produce and fresh animal products. Then we'll start to eliminate food products that encourage the growth of yeast. Among the greatest offenders (and those you absolutely must avoid) are

- sugar and all sugar substitutes, including sugar alcohols and artificial sweeteners
- brewer's yeast
- baked goods that use yeast in their preparation process, including bread, pastries, rolls, and pretzels
- alcoholic drinks that have been fermented, including beer, wine, brandy, whiskey, rum, cider, and homemade alcoholic beverages with the exception of vodka and gin not more than once a week
- vinegar and foods containing vinegar (with the exception of apple cider vinegar, which is not yeast-producing), including most pickles, most commercial mayonnaise, mincemeat, horseradish, and ketchup
- certain condiments, including soy sauce, Worcestershire sauce, steak sauce, and chutneys
- pickled and smoked meats
- mushrooms and truffles
- dairy products, including cheese, sour cream, buttermilk, cottage cheese, and cream cheese
- dried and candied fruits
- fruit juice
- melons

- excessive fruits (note that for the first two weeks of the 21-day program we will be eliminating all fruits)
- excessive canned tomatoes or tomato juice (homemade is OK)
- any supplements that are yeast-based (check labels)

Phase out pharmaceuticals that support yeast growth. Certain prescription drugs can encourage overgrowth of yeast, including steroids, birth control pills, and antibiotics. Always consult your doctor before you discontinue medication, but if you're already taking these, or your doctor recommends them, talk to him or her about any possible alternatives.

Buttress your probiotic population during antibiotic treatments. If you must take antibiotics, then make sure to double up on your probiotics for at least three months. You can take probiotics two hours before or two hours after antibiotics. This is perhaps the most critical anti-yeast measure you can take.

Cut way back on carbs. Severely restrict sugar, refined grains, and even whole grains, that contain gluten, especially wheat, rye, and barley. Sugar is undoubtedly yeast's favorite food, but both refined and even whole gluten-containing grains can stimulate yeast overgrowth. Better choices on an anti-yeast regimen include rice, quinoa, buckwheat, millet, and amaranth. Note: We'll talk more about the specific recommendations for a yeast-proof diet in later chapters, but for now, focus on these broader guidelines.

Have some garlic every day. Research in India has shown that garlic paste can be as effective as prescription medicines in suppressing oral Candida infections. Allicin, the ingredient in garlic that provides its distinctive flavor, also acts as a natural fungicide. If you take garlic supplements, make sure they contain allicin. Alternatively, eat one to two garlic cloves per day in your food.

Take probiotic supplements. As part of your Gut Flush Plan, you're already taking probiotics. This is where quality really comes in. Dr. Ohhira's Probiotics 12 PLUS contains twelve strains of live lactic acid bacteria, ten vitamins, eight minerals, and eighteen amino acids. The most crucial ingredient is E. faecalis TH10, a special strain of lactic acid–producing bacteria. Research demonstrates that this TH10 type of bacteria may also help protect against intestinal anthrax, E. coli, H. pylori, and antibiotic-resistant Superbugs.

Compensate for yeast's nutritional thievery. According to Leo Galland, M.D., assistant clinical professor at the University of Connecticut Health Center, yeast infections influence the manner in which the body metabolizes certain vitamins and minerals. When yeast actively overgrows, nutrient deficiencies may occur simultaneously. For example, yeast has been shown to increase the level of magnesium your body excretes, but you can compensate by eating more green vegetables, nuts (with the exception of peanuts that are often contaminated with aflatoxin), and seafood. Vitamin B6 may suffer the same fate; offset with avocados, gluten-free grains, and walnuts. Also, get more biotin, a B vitamin that stops yeast from shifting into an aggressive stage; good sources are egg yolks, legumes, and nuts. I personally recommend a biotin supplement like the Biotin 5 mg (see Resources). And as always, consult a knowledgeable health practitioner or nutritionist for specific recommendations for your individual needs.

Try Pau d'Arco. An herbal tea also known as Taheebo, Pau d'Arco is an antifungal. It can be purchased in bulk or as individual bags in health food stores.

Use oil of oregano. This natural substance is made form wild oregano, a plant that grows in sparsely populated, remote mountainous areas free of pollution. The oil is extracted naturally without the use of chemicals or solvents. The strength of this oil as a potent germ killer led Jean Valnet, in his seminal work, *The Practice of Aromatherapy,* to note that it can even sterilize sewage. A study in the *International Journal of Food Microbiology* showed that oil of oregano is an effective germicide that can kill a wide spectrum of fungi and bacteria. Other research in the *Journal of Applied Nutrition* shows that it can kill Candida. Scientists in Mexico have found that oil of oregano works against parasites and is particularly effective against Giardia. I recommend the liquid oil made by the North American Herb & Spice Company. Take five drops two to three times per day in water.

Try some additional Gut Flush Anti-Yeast Supplements. Supplements that promote healthy intestinal flora and support the body's anti-yeast defenses are crucial for long-term maintenance of an internal environment that resists Candida. The supplements that follow are based upon formulations that I have used with my own clients and have suggested to my readers for years. They are available directly from Uni Key or you can locate similar formulations in health food stores or online.

- **Y-C Cleanse.** This homeopathic formula is clinically shown to be safe and effective against Candida albicans and other yeast overgrowth that may cause allergies, bloating, fatigue, food cravings, and other discomforts. Y-C Cleanse is designed for both acute symptoms and maintenance. The product should be taken for at least twenty-four days with a five- or six-day break; then resume treatment if symptoms persist.
- **Flora Key.** This powdered intestinal flora formula, along with Dr. Ohhira's Probiotics 12 PLUS, supports a healthy intestinal environment. This probiotic contains acidophilus, bifidus, and fructooligosaccharides (FOS), which makes it an ideal Gut Flush sweetener and a convenient way to take probiotics if you don't like swallowing pills. Use about one teaspoon per day instead of sugar in no-heat recipes. Each teaspoon of Flora Key powder contains 6.5 billion active organisms.
- **Female Multiple Vitamin.** This is an all-in-one copper-free supplement I have designed to fulfill a woman's special needs. Formulated to be safe for both pregnant and breast-feeding women (with 800 mcg of folic acid), this supplement contains twice as much magnesium as calcium, a ratio that optimizes calcium absorption for strong bones and relaxed muscles. The Female Multiple supports balanced hormone levels for women of any age. The plant-based enzymes promote absorption of all the essential female vitamins, minerals, antioxidants, and phytonutrients. Take two capsules three times per day with meals.
- **Formula SF 722.** This yeast fighter contains undecenoic acid, derived from castor bean oil. This has been a remarkably successful formula with many of my clients with hard-to-eradicate Candida. Take one to two capsules two to three times daily with or between meals.

Now we'll turn to our fearsome Colon Corruptor #2: parasites. You may not be able to always see them, but I bet you are going to feel them when you read what's ahead. Chances are, they're making themselves at home inside of you right now. Turn to the next chapter to find out how they got inside you, how you can detect them, and exactly how the Gut Flush Plan will help you start to evict them.

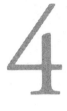

Colon Corruptor #2:
Parasites

Parasite. The very word can make you squirm with discomfort.

Mention parasites and many people picture Third World countries where dirty creeks drain off sewage and garbage. But the idea of parasite infestation as a far-flung problem is way out of date. One study found that one of every three Americans who submitted fecal samples for examination tested positive for parasites. That means, statistically, it's almost certain that you or somebody in your family has a parasitic infection, whether or not it's causing you Gut Grief.

The problem is real and growing more critical every year. Consider these cases:

- In 1993, in Milwaukee, Cryptosporidium in tap water caused 403,000 cases of acute gastrointestinal disease. Cryptosporidium resists standard water treatment and is so problematic that the CDC has identified it as a category B pathogen—something that could be used as a bioterrorist weapon.
- In 1996, about fourteen hundred Americans were infected with the parasite cyclospora after eating raspberries imported from Guatemala. Re-

searchers believe the water used to spray fungicides on the raspberries was probably contaminated with infected feces.

- In 2006, scientists found evidence suggesting that parasites make us fat! Researchers at Penn State uncovered a metabolic problem among the dragonfly population that looks eerily similar to the obesity epidemic in humans. These dragonflies harbored parasites similar to those that cause malaria and cryptosporidiosis. As a result, they experienced inflammation that impeded their metabolism of fat, resulting in increased fat accumulation fat around their muscles. Researchers believe that similar parasitic developments in humans may be partly responsible for the human epidemics of insulin resistance, type 2 diabetes, and obesity.

We are exposed to parasites daily. I am talking about those microscopic organisms to foot-long tapeworms that can eventually take up residence in your body. In fact, some experts say North Americans are exposed to more parasites than people in other parts of the world. All signs indicate that parasites represent a greatly underestimated threat to everyone's health. If we learn nothing else, let's take a lesson from the dragonflies: we must flush our digestive systems of parasites if we want to lose our body fat and get healthy.

Worming Their Way into You

Parasites are responsible for several common symptoms of Gut Grief, but they're also a vastly underacknowledged source of many other health problems. As I discussed in my book *Guess What Came to Dinner?*, I was first made aware of our parasitic health problem back in 1974 when Hazel Parcells, D.C., N.D., Ph.D., made the situation clear in a class about "scientific nutrition" in Albuquerque, New Mexico. In that lecture, Dr. Parcells provided unforgettable bottled samples of the repulsive worms and other undesirables that often dwell in the human digestive tract. Her main point: parasites are the unrecognized cause of not only digestive discomforts but also many diseases that seem unrelated to the digestive tract. Conditions that are linked to parasites can certainly appear identical to those that are connected to Candida and a lack of beneficial bacteria because all three can be found in the same out-of-balance internal environment. These conditions can include, but are not restricted to:

- constipation
- diarrhea
- gas and bloating
- infecto-obesity
- allergies
- asthma
- persistent flulike symptoms
- chronic fatigue
- unexplained joint and muscle aches and pains
- immune problems
- anemia
- secondary gluten and lactose intolerance
- irritable bowel syndrome
- Crohn's disease
- skin conditions
- nervous system disorders
- teeth grinding
- sleep disturbances
- enlarged liver or spleen

The problem is that the average physician and clinical laboratory are often unable to diagnose parasite problems. In a study of diagnostic labs in the United States, researchers found that only about one in ten facilities could correctly identify cases of amebic dysentery, a parasite that kills up to one hundred thousand people worldwide every year. Most medical practitioners are unaware that parasites are frequently the root causes of a host of health problems.

And just where are these parasites finding us? The short answer is—everywhere.

Risk Factors for Parasite Infestation

Parasites inhabit our bodies, suck up our nutrients and our health reserves, sap our energy, and often block vital organs. You can pick up anything from a one-celled organism to worms and other larger creatures from food and water. But these days, parasites can strike due to a variety of factors in the environment. Basically any time you're in a public place, you can pick up parasites—you are rarely safe from their reach. Even as you read this, your defenses against the parasites that inhabit the world around you are being tested, probed, and breached.

Day-care settings. Just the single parasite Giardia can cause chronic fatigue, persistent diarrhea, bloating, cramps, flatulence, and unintentional weight loss. This microscopic organism is notorious for being passed around at day-care centers, as well as being found in lakes, rivers, and streams. If you have a child in day care, make sure he or she washes her hands all the time—research shows Giardia can frequent day-care center counters, sinks, and chairs.

Travel. The world we live in gets smaller every year: intercontinental jet travel is now common for millions of people. Each year more than 700 million passengers ride airplanes. While less than half of all Americans rode in commercial jets in 1975, today more than 80 percent use air transportation. Mankind's increasing mobility is one of the best-known reasons for the parasite crisis.

Plenty of people bring back parasites from other countries. About one hundred cases of dengue fever occur every year in tourists coming back to the United States. At the same time, schistosomiasis, a parasitic worm, infects 200 million people worldwide and can cause anemia, chronic pain, diarrhea, fatigue, and poor absorption of nutrients. You might pick up this particular worm after an otherwise innocent swim in contaminated water.

And just as parasites can infect your gut and your skin, they can infect the outer shell of an airplane. Studies now show that deadly microorganisms don't even have to get inside the plane to hop a ride. These hardy bugs can attach to the outside metal of a jet fuselage and actually survive an intercontinental trip—and arrive safe and sound in the United States and still be infectious. That's why its important to know how and where to get checked when strange symptoms like sudden high fevers come to call.

Global warming. Atmospheric changes brought on by technology, cars, and manufacturing have generally warmed the air, allowing parasites and other infectious organisms to survive in greater numbers and expand their range. Changes in ocean currents have upset the ecological balance of the seas, and scientists believe that warming temperatures and extra flooding due to climate change will lead to significant increases in mosquitoes and other insects that convey parasites. A recent EPA report warned that global warming may soon bring dengue, passed on by mosquitoes, to the United States. Dengue's devastating effects include intense joint pain, severe headaches, and muscle pains.

Imported foods. Our supermarkets are now gathering places for foods from around the world. Many of those items have not been properly inspected before being brought into the country and sold. And when they are inspected, the results are disturbing: from July 2006 to July 2007, the U.S. Food and Drug Administration sent back more than nineteen hundred shipments of food and cosmetics from China because they were contaminated. At the same time, the agency also rejected more than seventeen hundred shipments from India and fifteen hundred shipments from Mexico.

Huge, centralized food companies. Contamination becomes a big problem when much of our food comes from big manufacturers. Today, an individual hamburger contains the meat of one hundred cows. Consequently, when one animal is contaminated, the chance of a large amount of food being contaminated increases dramatically. That's why food recalls are often so widespread—the meat of that one cow could be on tables all over the country. Consider ConAgra's 2002 recall of *19 million pounds* of hamburger. Or Castleberry's 2007 recall of *721,389 pounds* of canned meat products distributed in Alabama, New York, California, Connecticut, Georgia, and seventeen other states across North America. Now more than ever you have a great reason to buy locally produced foods.

Increased development of land. Housing developments mean more pollution and more stress on natural ecosystems. Scientists now know that even rainfall patterns have been distorted by the development of cities. By the year 2025, it is estimated, 70 percent of the world's population will live in cities and suburbs. This increased crowding and resulting environmental changes mean more parasite epidemics and infectious diseases.

Restaurant dining. Our penchant for eating out has meant a big boost in food-borne illness. Local restaurants have little oversight other than random checks from the health department. Some franchises of corporate fast-food chains emphasize "efficiency" over cleanliness, and minimum wage fast-food workers on bathroom breaks are pressured to get back to work quickly, sometimes at the expense of good hygiene. The mere fact that food chains put such great emphasis on profits and doing a large volume of business means that customers' health may be at greater risk.

Raw and undercooked fruits and vegetables. The CDC estimates that four of five pathogenic outbreaks are linked to food and water. Sadly, even eating what's frequently considered a healthy diet, one filled with raw fruits and vegetables, can put you at greater risk. When you eat raw foods, you grant parasites entry into the body's inner spaces where they happily prosper. Clinging to the peels of fruits, hidden among leaves of lettuce, floating in smoothies, and lurking in cuts of meat, parasites are always seeking passage into your body where they can be nourished and reproduce at your expense. Research in Europe shows that if Cryptosporidium gets on a leaf of lettuce, 10 percent of the parasite population will survive three full days of refrigeration. Berries, cherries, raspberries, strawberries, bamboo shoots, water chestnuts, watercress, spinach, parsley, lettuce, and celery are frequent homes to parasites unless, of course, you are washing the produce in the special Gut Flush Food Bath discussed in Chapter 3.

Raw and undercooked beef. You should never eat raw beef (also known as steak tartare or thin-sliced carpaccio among gourmets). Beef can be a source of tapeworm, a particularly sneaky parasite that dwells inside you without causing symptoms. Rare burgers or steaks are also risky. They can contain a single-celled parasite called toxoplasmosis that is also found in cat feces. This parasite can cause birth defects and encephalitis. All beef needs to be cooked to an internal temperature of 160 degrees Fahrenheit to ensure the destruction of parasites.

Pork. Pork can be the source of the well-known parasite trichinosis. Pigs pick up trichinosis from contaminated garbage or infected rodents. If you eat infected pork, the parasites' encysted larvae hatch in the intestines and then move to muscle tissue. In the process it causes flulike symptoms and excruciating muscle aches and pains.

Improperly prepared ham, sausage, and pork can also be infected with pork tapeworm. This worm can cause serious brain damage because its larvae often migrate into brain tissue.

Because of these infestations in pork, the "other white meat" should never be prepared in a microwave oven. Microwaves don't heat food evenly, leaving parts of the pork cold enough to let parasites survive. Pork should be cooked in a conventional oven (or on the stove top) so that its internal temperature reaches 170 degrees Fahrenheit.

Fish. Fish are another rich source of parasites, providing homes to flukes, fish tapeworms, and anisakine larvae. The tapeworms found in raw salmon can cause anemia when they monopolize your vitamin B_{12} and are also linked to nervous system problems. Be aware that the type of cut is very important—salmon fillets are less often contaminated than salmon steaks. The steaks are made from the fish's abdominal area, a part of the fish that can be teeming with worms. Other fish that can be infected with tapeworms include turbot, pike, lake trout, perch, orange roughy, and grayling.

Anisakine nematode larvae are found in cod, herring, Pacific salmon, and red snapper. If you eat fish infested with surviving anisakine, the larvae drill into the stomach or intestinal wall, causing devastating pain. The resulting symptoms resemble appendicitis, gastric ulcers, and stomach cancer. When infestations get bad enough, infected sections of a patient's intestines may have to be surgically removed. For the same reasons, you shouldn't cook pork in a microwave; don't use a microwave to cook fish, either. It may be all right for reheating, but that's only after it has been cooked in a conventional oven.

Tap water. When he said "In wine there is wisdom, in beer there is freedom, in water there is bacteria," Benjamin Franklin may have been trying to rationalize his fondness for alcohol, but the sage philosopher is quite right about this one. Tap water is a shaky bet, at best. According to researchers, more than a million Americans a year contract gastrointestinal illness from bad water, and about a thousand die. Because our climate is getting warmer and we're using up more and more water, our municipal water supplies are being pushed to their limits and often can't keep up with the parasite crisis. One of the most serious parasites found in water is Giardia, which the CDC has identified as the most frequent cause of waterborne disease. As I mentioned before, Giardia can cause bloating, foul flatulence, diarrhea, nausea, intestinal irritation, and cramps that last for weeks, months, or years. For safety's sake, the CDC recommends that those with compromised immunity, senior citizens, and pregnant women should always boil their water. Bottled water is unregulated and therefore unreliable as a pure source of water for those with comprised or sensitive systems.

Dogs and cats. While your pet may be your best friend, he may also be the source of your parasites. Experts estimate that you can catch more than thirty illnesses from your pet. Admittedly, a dog can boost your health by soothing your spirit and keeping you company—but just know that all puppies are born infected with a dog roundworm called Toxocara canis. Half of all dogs may harbor parasites like hookworms, tapeworms, heartworms, and roundworms, and any park, road, lawn, or outdoor area frequented by dogs can be infested with parasites transmitted in dog feces. Researchers have found that up to 20 percent of soil in parks and playgrounds contains Toxocara from dogs.

Cats are also a source of parasites. They pass on Toxoplasma gondii, a parasite in their feces that can cause birth defects and symptoms that resemble mononucleosis and lymphatic disorders. That's why pregnant women shouldn't even think about going near a kitty litter box.

BLOCK PARASITES AT THE DOOR

Parasites are all around us, itching to get into our bodies—but we don't have to let them. Try these strategies to keep parasites out.

- Wash your hands for twenty seconds before preparing food or eating (a study published in *The Lancet* showed that proper hand washing can reduce the incidence of diarrhea by 50 percent).
- Wash your hands after handling pets, changing diapers, or using the bathroom.
- Keep your fingernails short and scrubbed.
- Always wipe toilet seats before you sit.
- Never use tap water to clean contact lenses.
- Never walk barefoot outdoors.
- If you travel frequently, often eat at restaurants, have pets, or live in or near mountains, be tested for parasites at least twice a year.

The fleas carried by dogs and cats can spread tapeworms if you unwittingly ingest these insects. Plus, pets can be Giardia and Cryptosporidium carriers after they drink contaminated water or contact infected feces. Bottom line: step lively, wear gloves when you clean up after your pet, wash your hands frequently, and stay current with your pet's health care.

Do You Have Parasites?

All right, it's now obvious that parasites are all around us right here in the good ol' USA. That's bad enough. But when you factor in the reality that parasites are the "great masqueraders," it can really be frustrating to figure out what is really going on with your body. Giardia can cause chronic fatigue or irritable bowel syndrome. A case of roundworms can seem like an allergy and asthma. Pinworms can be the source of your child's hyperactivity. Amoeba can be mistaken for ulcerative colitis. But few medical doctors are aware or even suspect that there could be a parasite link when symptoms don't resolve.

Usually, the way parasites have been diagnosed is with a stool study. But even this method may prove unreliable. If a parasite like trichinosis lives in your blood or in your muscles, how are you going to find it in your stool? You won't. Others, like pinworms or dogworms, may not be accommodating enough to show up during your lab test. Those that cling to the walls of the gastrointestinal tract also stay out of feces.

When parasites are passed out through bowel movements, they may show up on some days but not on others. Parasite detection requires persistence. In many cases, it can take up to nine stool samples to find evidence of parasites. This questionnaire can indicate the probability that you are infected with parasites, especially if you have tried other treatments to no avail.

APPARENT SYMPTOMS
Are you often very tired?
Does your eyesight sometimes get blurry?
Do food cravings often make you prone to binge eating?
Do you have breathing difficulties?
Do you get ringing in your ears?
Is your skin yellow?
Have you had continual diarrhea?
Do meals leave you unsatisfied and still hungry?
Do your lips often turn blue?
Have you had rectal and anal itchiness that won't go away?
Do you have bloating and intestinal gas after meals?
Are you plagued by stomach pain and cramps?
Have you been diagnosed with anemia?
Do you have persistent insomnia?
Does you weight yo-yo up and down for no reason?
Do you experience frequent patches of itchy skin or rashes?
Do you suffer frequent allergic reactions?
Do you have a problem with grinding your teeth?
Are you often constipated?
Do you have very many, varied sex partners?

TRAVEL HISTORY
Have you ever experienced mysterious symptoms after a trip?
Have you been overseas to Asia, Africa, Europe, Central America, South
    America, or Mexico?
Have you ever visited or do you live in Hawaii?
Do you go on hikes and/or swim in rivers, lakes, streams, reservoirs, or rock
    quarries?

INSIDE AND AROUND YOUR HOME
Do you live on or near a farm?

Does your drinking water come from a well?

Do you consume a large amount of raw foods?

Does your family eat meat that is very rare?

Do you have a pet, such as a cat or dog, that goes both indoors and out?

Do you or other family members frequently forget to wash your hands after touching a pet?

Do you neglect to wash your hands before working in the kitchen?

Do you often use your microwave for cooking?

Do you or other family members forget to clean kitchen counters and cutting boards after cutting up raw meat?

DIET
Do you eat sushi?

Do you eat pork hot dogs?

Do you eat at salad bars?

Do you eat raw fruits and vegetables?

Do you eat dishes prepared by neighbors and friends at potluck suppers?

WORK HISTORY
Do you work in a hospital or doctor's office?

Do you work in a veterinary office?

Are you employed in child care?

Do you work in the sanitation department?

Have you ever been in the military and assigned overseas duty?

Do you perform farm work?

CHILDREN'S SYMPTOMS
Do any of your children have trouble sleeping?

Do any of your children bleed for no apparent reason?

Do any of your children wet the bed?

Have you noticed dark circles under any of your children's eyes?

Are any of your children short for their ages or too thin?

Do your children cough for no apparent reason?

Does your baby cry all the time?

Does your baby repetitively bang her head?

Does your baby suffer persistent colic?

Does your baby have a rash around her diaper?

For adults: If a dozen or more of these are true for you, you may have a significant risk for parasites.

For children and infants: If any of these apply, ask your doctor about testing your children for parasites.

The Gut Flush Antiparasite Protocol

If you have parasites, you need professional help in getting rid of them. A health care practitioner with the proper background in treating parasites is essential. Also, remember that if one family member has parasites, all family members should be treated. Otherwise reinfection may occur from a silent carrier of the parasite.

Treating parasites requires getting to the root cause of the problem, not just alleviating the symptoms. Of course, if the symptoms are life threatening, as when a person with AIDS or another immunity-compromising condition is suffering dehydrating diarrhea from a parasite, putting an immediate stop to the symptom is essential. Talk to your experienced health care practitioner about incorporating these suggestions into your antiparasite protocol.

Continue your Gut Flush Basic Protocol. Each of the elements of the protocol—probiotics, HCl, and digestive enzymes—are critical to the process of parasite elimination. Make sure that you begin with the loading dose of the probiotics, five capsules twice a day, but extend the basic protocol suggestion by two days, for up to a full week. Then switch to the maintenance dose of two capsules twice a day. Take your doses on an empty stomach—first thing in the morning and last thing at night before going to bed. Continue to take your HCl and digestive enzymes with each meal.

Limit raw foods of all kinds, especially if you eat out. Eat plenty of properly cooked proteins like fish, meat, chicken, and eggs. Protein provides the amino acids necessary to strengthen tissues and enhance immunity. To eliminate parasites on the home front, bathe all produce and proteins in the Gut Flush Food Bath described in Chapter 3.

Gently increase fiber intake. We'll be talking about the wondrous Fortifying and Flushing power of both soluble and insoluble fiber extensively throughout the Gut Flush Plan. For now, work on increasing your fiber intake to at least 25 grams per day. My clients have told me that it takes time for their bodies to adapt to a higher fiber diet and that is very difficult to get even the minimum 25 grams of fiber on a cleansing diet with their sensitive GI tracts. For these reasons, I usually recommend a fiber-based supplement like the Super-GI Cleanse (see below) which contains five sources of the least-irritating soluble and insoluble fibers such as oat bran, rice bran, apple pectin, ground flaxseed, and psyllium. Vegetarians should cut back on excessive amounts of beans, nuts, seeds, peas, and legumes which may simply be too much for the GI tract at this time.

Limit sugars and highly processed carbs. A diet high in simple carbohydrates like sugar, white flour, processed foods, and milk can fuel your uninvited guests. Even so-called "natural sweets"—honey, barley malt, fruit, fruit juice sweeteners, and concentrates—taken in excess can provide instant nourishment for your internal hitchhikers. Eating fiber-deficient foods may have been what attracted these parasites to your internal environment to begin with. Simple carbohydrate foods require more time to pass through the alimentary system. A sluggish transit time allows more food to decay and putrefy, thus producing stagnation in the colon and an inviting environment for toxic buildup.

Eliminate cold drinks. These act as a shock to the body and cause the intestinal tract to contract and hold on to waste materials, exactly what you don't want during this detox period.

Avoid most dairy and gluten-based products. Many parasites, like roundworm and Giardia, can precipitate secondary lactose (milk sugar) intolerance, so avoiding milk and cheese is a must. The exception to this dairy ban would be plain organic yogurt and kefir. In these products, milk sugar is fermented into healthy lactic acid rich in enzymes and live microorganisms that provide natural probiotics. Butter and cream are also exceptions to this rule as they are fats and digested differently.

Because of the damaged intestinal villi, Giardia can also produce gluten intolerance—the inability to digest the protein portion of wheat and rye and to a lesser extent barley. With any protozoan infection that can damage the intestinal villi, it is always a good idea to reduce the intake of grains.

Up the beta-carotene. Based upon clinical studies it appears that of all the vitamins and minerals, vitamin A best increases resistance to tissue penetration by parasitic larvae. Foods rich in pre-vitamin A or beta-carotene (think brightly colored orange and green veggies) should be added liberally to the diet. This is why the 21-Day Gut Flush Plan includes foods rich in beta-carotene.

Think zinc. Along with vitamin A–rich foods, please increase your zinc. Vitamin A and zinc are by far the two most important nutrients to add to your diet for parasite-proofing. Zinc can be found in beef, turkey, lamb, eggs, and pumpkin seeds.

Use onions, garlic, cloves, and fennel in cooking. These are all well-respected and time-honored parasite controllers.

Try colonic cleansing. Home enemas and colonic irrigation can play an important role in cleansing the colon of parasites. Garlic enemas, for example, are especially helpful in eliminating pinworms. We'll talk about these methods more extensively in Chapter 8. (See page 116 for more information on colonics.)

Take a tablespoon of fish and flaxseed oils. A key part of the Fortify section of the Gut Flush Plan involves omega-3 fatty acids (see page 98 in Chapter 7 for more information). I've found that fish and flaxseed oils are especially helpful with parasites because their fatty acids are absorbed so readily in the structure of the body's cellular membranes thus providing protection down to the cellular level against hidden invaders. The oils also lubricate the gastrointestinal tract and serve as a carrier for fat-soluble vitamin A, creating an environment uninviting for waste, toxins, and microorganism buildup.

Sip therapeutic teas. Drink one to two cups of mugwort tea every day. Mugwort hardly sounds like a serious name, but the tea made from this herb has been used for generations to kill intestinal parasites. (We'll talk more about mugwort in Chapter 8.)

Try some additional Gut Flush Antiparasite Supplements. Supplements that promote gentle cleansing of the colon will typically help reduce the number of intestinal parasites. The supplements that follow are based upon formulations that I have used with my own clients and have suggested to my readers for years. They are available directly from Uni Key or you can locate similar formulations in health food stores or online. Consider adding some of these additional supplements to speed the cleansing process:

- *Super-GI Cleanse.* In my opinion, this is one of the best products on the market to accomplish successful Gut Flushing (see Resources). Here are some special features of the key ingredients:
  - Cranberry powder, a substance rich in organic acids that appear to function as natural digestive enzymes to assist in the elimination of parasites and worms from every organ, tissue, and system, especially the lymphatics. Cranberry powder also helps with pH balance—so critical in protecting us from becoming a breeding ground for microorganisms, yeast, and other toxins.
  - Psyllium seed husk fiber, the "carbohydrate gum" found in the cell wall of psyllium, known for its ability to absorb water and speed bowel transit time.
  - Flaxseed fiber, an abundant source of lignan precursors, which exhibit properties such as anticancer, antibacterial, antifungal, and antiviral activity.
  - Apple pectin, the gel-forming properties of which are responsible for lowering cholesterol by binding the cholesterol and bile acids in the gut and promoting their excretion.
  - Alfalfa leaves, high in saponins, which help to reduce serum cholesterol levels and possibly reverse atherosclerotic plaque.
  - Butternut root bark, known for ages as one of the safest and mildest laxatives while helping in the secretion of bile. Also helps to prevent and ward off worms.
  - Fennel seed, a natural digestive aid that helps to eliminate flatulence.
  - Peppermint leaves, used for centuries to aid digestion, absorb intestinal gas, inhibit constipation and diarrhea, and stimulate the secretion of bile. Peppermint also has the ability to fight off and eliminate microorganisms such as parasites, influenza, and many other viruses.

- Irish moss, a bulk laxative that soothes and coats the complete GI tract and helps eliminate heavy metals.
- Licorice root, a protector and healer of irritated mucous membranes that also supports adrenal gland function.
- Aniseed, an antispasmodic that helps eradicate bloating and gas.
- A special enzyme blend that targets digestion of protein, carbohydrates, and fat.
- A probiotic blend that enhances immunity and helps with the absorption of the B vitamins and vitamin K.

- *My Colon Cleansing Kit.* This thirty-day program provides advanced, safe, and gentle colon cleansings, while targeting accumulated waste, microorganisms, and toxins to increase energy, nutrient absorption, and overall colon health. It includes three time-tested and unique herbal products designed to help eliminate parasites while recolonizing your system with friendly probiotics to promote a clean colon, immunity, and healthy digestion. It includes Para-Key™, Verma-Plus™, and Flora-Key™. I recommend you use the kit for thirty days. If you still have gas or feel bloated after the initial thirty days, you may want to consider continuing for another thirty days. Do not use this kit during pregnancy or while nursing.

Directions for My Colon Cleansing Kit:

Weeks One & Two:

Para-Key™: Take two capsules, three times daily twenty to thirty minutes before meals.

Verma-Plus™: Take one dropper (twenty-seven drops or one-quarter teaspoon), two times daily in four ounces of water between meals on an empty stomach and once at bedtime.

Flora-Key™: Take one teaspoon daily with six to eight ounces of water on an empty stomach.

Rest five days.

Weeks Three & Four:

Para-Key™: Take two capsules, three times daily twenty to thirty minutes before meals.

Verma-Plus™: Take one dropper (twenty-seven drops or one-quarter teaspoon), two times daily in four ounces of water between meals on an empty stomach and once at bedtime.

Flora-Key™: Take one teaspoon daily with six to eight ounces of water on an empty stomach.

- *Para-Key*™. An herbal formula consisting of cranberry concentrate, grapefruit seed extract, artemisia annua, garlic, cayenne, slippery elm, and bromelain. Take two capsules, three times daily twenty to thirty minutes before meals or as directed by a health care professional. For children forty to eighty pounds, take half the adult dosage. Not recommended for children under forty pounds.*

- *Verma-Plus*™. A liquid herbal tincture that cleanses the GI tract of larger organisms and toxins for optimal health and function. One full dropper (twenty-seven drops or one-quarter teaspoon) contains: Proprietary Blend—1.25 mL, black walnut, wormwood, centaury, male fern, orange peel, cloves, butternut. Take one full dropper (twenty-seven drops or one-quarter teaspoon), in four ounces of water between meals on an empty stomach and once at bedtime or as directed by a health care professional. For children forty to eighty pounds, take half the adult dosage. Not recommended for children under forty pounds.*

- *Flora-Key*™. This Gut Flushing sweetener recommended in the Gut Flush Plan is a potent probiotic in its own right. It is very compatible with the probiotic formula discussed in chapters 2 and 3. One teaspoon contains: Lactobacillus acidophilus, Bifidobacterium bifidum, Bifidobacterium longum—650 mg. Microflora Growth Concentrate FOS (Fructo-oligosaccharides—Minimum Concentration 96 percent)—2,400 mg.

*For children under forty pounds, I usually recommend a product called Zymex II, which can be opened up and mixed in water or foods if necessary. Two capsules twice per day between meals is usually the recommended dosage. I would start with one capsule and increase slowly. This product contains natural digestive enzymes and extracts from figs and almonds. It is highly effective for pinworms (see Resources).

Take one teaspoon mixed in six to eight ounces of water on an empty stomach once per day or as directed by a health care professional. For children forty to eighty pounds, take half the adult dosage.

In the next chapter, we'll take on Colon Corruptor #3, one that's been making a lot of headlines lately: Superbugs. They're all around us, but we don't have to be helpless victims—the Gut Flush Plan will arm you so you can defend yourself and your family from these terrifying and potentially deadly bacteria.

5

Colon Corruptor #3: Superbugs

A FIERY, BURNING SENSATION IN HER STOMACH HAD BOTHERED WANDA for years, but she just ignored it and endured the discomfort. She thought it was the price she had to pay for working at a high-pressure job as the manager of the children's clothing department. The constant hassles in dealing with employees, buyers, corporate management, and manufacturers seemed to incite her ulcer into a volcanic internal inferno. So she gulped down an endless supply of antacids and kept working through the pain.

Until, that is, her Gut Grief caught up with her. One day at work, she leaned over to pick up a box of dresses and became dangerously light-headed. The dizziness and queasiness got so bad, she couldn't stand back up.

When she got to the hospital, she was rushed into the emergency room. After an endoscopy, the doctor came back to her bedside to deliver the news. "Wanda, you have a bleeding ulcer," he said. "Had you not come in today, there was a good chance you would have died."

It took a week of hospitalization and five pints of blood to get Wanda back on her feet. Meanwhile, further tests revealed that the Superbug that had caused Wanda's ulcer—H. pylori—had spread to her teenage son and daughter. "I was shocked," says Wanda now. "I thought only adults could get ulcers."

To stem this outbreak of ulcers, Wanda and her children received two courses of what doctors call "triple therapy"—a simultaneous treatment with three types of antibiotics. (Of course, it goes without saying that this therapy also destroys the beneficial bacteria or probiotics in your digestive tract.)

Wanda eventually recovered from her ulcer and has since become a client of mine. She now protects herself naturally with the Gut Flush Plan and, thankfully, her pain hasn't come back. But her story should be a wake-up call to us all. Wanda's cavalier attitude about her ulcer was typical—and so were the complications that ulcers can cause when they're not taken seriously enough. Wanda almost died from her ulcer because she didn't understand the Superbug that had caused it and how dangerous this brand of Gut Grief can be.

Superbugs, bacteria that are resistant to almost all antibiotics, have been getting a lot of press lately. A 2007 *Journal of the American Medical Association* study about rapidly rising rate of fatalities linked to MRSA caused the whole nation to panic. Researchers had been warning about the risks of antibiotic resistance for years, but the study's revelations that this antibiotic-resistant strain of staph causes more than fifty deaths *every day* really drove the point home. To many, our vulnerability to Superbugs suddenly feels borderline cataclysmic.

You don't have to feel helpless. The truth is you *can* fight back. While the core Gut Flush Plan is designed to help give you the best possible resistance against all Superbugs, this chapter will help you devise a more targeted plan to prevent their infestation—or eradicate them, if they've already taken hold.

Knowledge is key, so we'll first take a look at a handful of very destructive Superbugs in our environment: Salmonella, E. coli, MRSA, and H. pylori. We'll spend the most time talking about H. pylori because, as Wanda's experience shows us, it's not only the cause of a common and painful manifestation of Gut Grief—the ulcer—it's also the most prevalent Superbug in the world. Let's find out if you're at risk for a Superbug infestation, what to do if you have one, and how to prevent one from ever gaining access to your gut.

Sneaky Salmonella

Since the late 1980s, one particular strain of Salmonella, Salmonella *Enteritidis,* has become the single most common cause of food poisoning in the United States. About six to forty-eight hours after you come into contact with Salmonella, you start to develop symptoms like nausea and vomiting; then, you may have stomach pains, a headache, fever, and/or diarrhea that can last another three or four days. Arthritic-type pains can become chronic three to four weeks after the onset of the more acute symptoms. For a full two months after you have this type of infection, you can still excrete Salmonella in your stools. That's why people who are carriers, especially food handlers who don't adequately wash their hands after going to the bathroom, can unwittingly spread this infection very easily.

The challenge is that you can't tell if Salmonella has contaminated food by looking at it, smelling it, or tasting it. Although the CDC says that most Salmonella originates in eggs, milk, poultry, and beef, we've seen deadly strains present themselves in peanut butter and unpasteurized fruit juice. The threat is serious and spreading fast.

Remember the story of Marty Jean from Chapter 1? Her horrific encounter with Salmonella, and the rest of the peanut butter Salmonella scares from 2006 and 2007, demonstrates one of the most frightening things about food contamination: often, government scientists have a hard time figuring out the point of origin. The processing of peanut butter requires high heat that is supposed to be hot enough to kill off Salmonella. The only explanation researchers could think of was that the peanut butter was put into dirty jars or was handled with contaminated equipment—but no one knows for sure. Despite the mystery, the bad peanut butter was found in thirty-nine states, made three hundred people sick, and sent about fifty to the hospital. Talk about Food Fright!

Here again is where gargantuan food manufacturers are a big part of the problem. Although supermarkets carry what seem to be a bewildering number of different brands of food, many of those are all made at the same factory. In the case of the peanut butter problem, it meant that several different brands were affected because they were all packaged at one plant. Similarly, when tainted ingredients show up in pet food, dozens of pet food brands have to be pulled from the shelves because the same manufacturer prepares so many brands.

And keep in mind, these stories are probably just the tip of the iceberg. Nobody knows how much is going unreported.

Salmonella is also found in pet feces and may be especially problematic in pets with diarrhea. Reptiles like pet turtles are especially prone to Salmonella, so kids who put their hands into their mouths may develop a Salmonella infection after handling animals. Children may also contract Salmonella from the animals at petting zoos. Luckily, the Gut Flush eating and lifestyle plan will help you prevent Salmonella from endangering your health and that of your family.

Icky E. Coli

E. coli is short for *Escherichia coli,* another group of bacteria that causes food poisoning. E. coli has been the reason behind the all too frequent recalls of hamburger meat and widespread problems with spinach. Just how problematic is E. coli? In 2007, a single recall of ground beef involved nearly 6 million pounds of meat in twenty-two states. When California bagged spinach was tainted with E. coli in the same year, it killed three people and made another two hundred sick.

Usually it takes about twenty-four to seventy-two hours after being infected to develop symptoms, which include abdominal pain, sudden (and severe) diarrhea, fever, gas, and cramps. Of course, you won't feel like eating much, but the good news is that you're not likely to vomit. With your run-of-the-mill E. coli infestation, most cases will resolve within three days. If you must endure E. coli infestation, that's the kind to get.

The worst cases of E. coli can be traced to a type known as E. coli O157:H7, a deadly pathogenic strain of the bug that has been found in raw meat but which can also contaminate spinach, green onions, lettuce, tomatoes, sprouts, melons, and other fruits and vegetables. This particular strain of E. coli is so toxic that a microscopic amount, as little as ten cells, can make you very sick and put you at death's door.

Once it's in your body, E. coli O157:H7 secretes a toxin that damages the small intestine, giving you cramps and bloody diarrhea that leave you dehydrated and exhausted. If your health is in decent shape, you should recover from the disease in about a week. But children, the elderly, and people with immune problems can suffer from what's called hemolytic uremic syndrome—severe kidney damage. Even with dialysis, this type of kidney failure can be fatal.

Changes in manufacturing processes, especially of hamburger, have made E. coli a much greater risk. Industrial grinding can transfer harmful bacteria from the meat's surface into the body of the hamburger. And contamination from a single cow can also compromise a staggering quantity of meat. For example, an average hamburger used to contain the meat of one or two cows; today, due to the industrial production of meat, a hamburger could contain the meat of *one hundred* cows. Bottom line: Superbugs love modern-day agribusiness because all of these practices help them gain wider access to an unsuspecting range of hosts.

Menacing MRSAs

Just as Superbugs are finding their way into our food, they're also devising other ways to enter our bodies and, of course, our GI systems. Take the most recent Superbug to sweep the nation: community-associated methicillin-resistant Staphylococcus aureus, or CA-MRSA.

Until 1998, MRSA infections were almost always connected to hospital stays. But somehow this infection has now spread beyond hospitals into schools, gyms, and salons. Since then, around the world, these types of pathogenic infections have frequently become "community-associated," which means they are found in everybody's neighborhood. In Chicago, for instance, the incidence of CA-MRSA increased more than sevenfold from the year 2000 to 2005.

Normally, this garden-variety staph is a harmless bacterium that lives on the skin or inside the noses of nearly one out of three people. But when you get bruised or nicked, this otherwise harmless bacterium can enter your skin and become particularly nasty. Once the bacteria gets under your skin, it can cause an abscess filled with pus in less than a day. While the infection usually stays near the surface, about 6 percent of the cases become invasive, entering the blood, destroying tissues, and attacking the heart and lungs.

Even healthy kids and athletes are not immune. A study of children's health in Texas found that CA-MRSA cases multiplied twelvefold between

2000 and 2003. In the spring of 2006, in Mountain Home, Arkansas, nine athletes and a coach were infected with CA-MRSA. Around the same time, a football player at the University of Tulsa named Devin Adair died of complications from CA-MRSA. Plus, Sammy Sosa, who was playing for the Baltimore Orioles in 2005, had to sit out more than a dozen games after a cut on his left foot became infected with CA-MRSA. Outbreaks of the infection have even closed down entire athletic departments.

Although you increase your chances of CA-MRSA if you've been in a hospital, play contact sports, frequent nail salons, use intravenous drugs, or have been tattooed, you can develop these serious infections from everyday shaving nicks, cuts, and abrasions, or bug bites. Still, there's hope against CA-MRSA, and the Gut Flush Plan can help you defend yourself and your family from this frightening epidemic.

Harmful H. pylori

Helicobacter bacteria got its name because its three tiny tails spin around and around like a helicopter. Outside the body, H. pylori is the most prevalent bacteria in the world, thought to infect three quarters of the world's population. In the body, H. pylori is linked to stomach and duodenal ulcers, heart disease, glaucoma, and even rosacea.

H. pylori often manages to outsmart the body. While GI Good Guy HCl kills off most harmful pathogens that try to enter the digestive tract, H. pylori shields itself from harm with a special enzyme named urease. Urease reacts

---

H. PYLORI: THE SUPERBUG THAT DESTROYS THE STOMACH

Your stomach and small intestine are lined with a layer of mucus that protects them from stomach acid and other liquids secreted into the digestive tract. Without this protection, which incorporates mucins, large proteins secreted on the surface, stomach acid would eat holes in the stomach and small intestine. When H. pylori compromises this protection, gaps are opened up that can lead to serious damage and injury. *(continued)*

When an ulcer forms, it allows stomach acid to enter the body and eat away at blood vessels and muscle tissue. That can cause serious bleeding. If this damage goes on too long, partially digested food and bacteria travel into your stomach cavity. This painful condition, called a perforated ulcer, leads to severe inflammation and requires surgery to correct. When ulcers form in the beginning of the small intestine (duodenum), this condition can totally block entry into the rest of the digestive tract. That situation also means you need surgery to fix the problem.

The most frequent sign that you have an ulcer is fiery, stabbing pain between your navel and breastbone right after you eat, although you can also feel pain on an empty stomach. Doctors generally diagnose ulcers by using an endoscopy (putting a tiny camera down your throat), a breath test, a blood test, or a test of a stool sample.

with waste material to produce ammonia that neutralizes HCl. Protected by this enzymatic process, H. pylori is free to proliferate and damage the protective lining of the stomach.

As the H. pylori increases, the stomach secretes extra acid to attack the invading bacteria. This extra acid does nothing to the H. pylori, as the bacteria is insulated from the acid's caustic effects. Instead, it creates gastritis, indigestion, heartburn, and sometimes leads to stomach cancer.

Taking antacids or drugs like ranitidine (Zantac) and cimetidine (Tagamet) may tamp down stomach acid, but those measures don't affect the H. pylori. What complicates the situation is the fact that neutralizing stomach acid may even contribute to the growth of even more H. pylori. (And, adding insult to already painful injury, long-term use of antacid drugs can cause diarrhea, constipation, stomach cramps, and even bone fractures due to the malabsorption of acid-requiring calcium.)

One way that we pick up H. pylori is from the feces of an infected person, another reason everyone should wash their hands frequently, scrubbing between the fingers and especially under the nails, after using the bathroom. It can also be conveyed in drinking water. One study by Penn State demonstrated a direct link between contaminated drinking water and stomach ulcers. The researchers pointed out that although water is tested for coliform,

ULCER MYSTERY SOLVED!

■

Though we now know that stomach ulcers are mostly caused by H. pylori, the medical establishment did not believe or acknowledge this key fact until it was proven by Australian researchers just two decades ago. Prior to that watershed discovery, ulcers had been the subject of more myths and false beliefs than just about any other illness. Doctors and researchers jumped to many wrong and often wildly strange conclusions.

A 1955 study at the University of Chicago by Lester R. Dragsted, M.D., a surgery professor, showed that ulcers are caused by a failure of the body's "telegraph system" to signal the brain to turn off gastric juices being delivered to the stomach. Dr. Dragsted insisted ulcers was an affliction visited upon those high up the corporate ladder.

In April 1960, ulcer expert H. Marvin Pollard, M.D., of the University of Michigan, spoke to a group of those business executives, claiming that just being "intense and intelligent" put you at risk for ulcers. This well-respected physician also believed that a man with ulcers (it was thought to be mostly a man's disease) "has not developed self-confidence [and] lacks faith in his own ability." But, Dr. Pollard reassured the crowd, men with ulcers "make good traveling companions." And while a few cigarettes a day were thought to be OK, the doctor warned against "excesses in smoking."

Ironically, a physician performing autopsies in the nineteenth century first noticed that bacteria in the stomach always seemed to be present when somebody died with ulcers. Throughout the twentieth century, doctors found evidence of these bacteria associated with ulcers, but they chalked it up to a mysterious form of contamination. They couldn't bring themselves to believe that this microorganism, H. pylori, caused the ulcers. If only they had drawn the right kind of conclusion.

another harmful bacterium, these tests often miss H. pylori. Drinking water dubbed "safe" may actually have rampant H. pylori.

H. pylori has made its share of headlines, too. In 2002, a group of researchers randomly went out shopping to a local grocery store and bought thirteen kinds of foods to evaluate for H. pylori. The results, reported at a conference of gastroenterologists in San Francisco, are disturbing. Forty percent of the chicken tested positive for H. pylori, and about one-third of the overall shrimp, pork, crab, clams, and fish were infected. Now we know why H. pylori is so prevalent worldwide!

While no one is sure why H. pylori seems to lead to ulcers in some people, when other people who have this bacteria never have these sorts of difficulties, the problem is probably one of balance. Those GI Good Guys, probiotics, that inhabit your digestive tract, help to keep H. pylori under control. Many studies show that taking probiotic bacteria can alleviate H. pylori complications.

Do You Have Superbugs?

Superbugs are diverse and devious, and detecting them is sometimes tricky. While we know that hospitals can be a dangerous place when it comes to picking up a staph infection, the Superbugs are now morphing into infections that are spreading in previously unsuspected locales like gyms, schools, and salons. When you learn how to spot and stop the Superbugs, you are well on your way to fighting back.

This questionnaire can indicate whether or not you are at significant risk of an infection by a Superbug that might resist treatment by the most common antibiotics.

OCCUPATIONAL HAZARDS

Do you work in construction, sanitation, or another occupation that runs a high risk of physical injury?

Does your work entail using instruments with sharp blades?

Do you work in a veterinary office?

Do you work as a health professional at a private medical practice?

Do you work in a hospital or long-term care facility?

Are you employed as a prison guard, or have you served time in prison?

Do you work in a restaurant where you frequently handle raw food?

PERSONAL FACTORS

Are you a high school, college, or professional athlete?

Are you African-American?

Are you female?

Are you under the age of forty?

Have you had multiple surgeries?

Do you frequently take antibiotics?

PERSONAL HABITS

Do you forget to wash your hands after going to the bathroom?

Do you forget to wash your hands after handling pets?

Do you neglect using gloves when doing yard work?

Have you used or do you currently use intravenous drugs?

Do you have a habit of picking your nose?

Do you eat raw, undercooked, or very rare meat?

Do you frequently dine at salad bars?

Do you consume more than two alcoholic drinks a day?

Have you been tattooed?

Do you have acrylic nails?

Do you get your cuticles cut or use a razor or grater on calluses?

ENVIRONMENTAL CONTRIBUTORS

Do you live in an overcrowded housing, such as a small apartment that is home to four or more people?

Do you live in public housing?

Do you live in a nursing home?

If you answer yes to two or more of these questions, you may indeed run a significant risk of contracting a Superbug infection.

The Gut Flush Anti-Superbug Protocol

Getting proper treatment for a Superbug can mean the difference between life and death, so if you have symptoms that lead you to suspect infestation, please see your doctor. A health care practitioner with the proper background in treating Superbugs is essential. Also, remember that if one family member has Superbugs, all family members should be treated. Otherwise you may trade the Superbug back and forth, as happened with Wanda and her family.

Many of the suggestions in the Gut Flush Anti-Superbug Protocol will center on prevention. One exception is H. pylori infestation resulting in ulcers—that is one condition that Gut Flush can help treat as well as prevent. (I'll note those suggestions that are especially helpful to ulcers below.)

Continue to take your Gut Flush Basic Protocol. In particular, make sure your probiotic contains bacterial strains known to destroy the Super-

---

KEEP SUPERBUGS AT BAY

Fighting the risk of Superbugs is an ongoing battle. When you're out in the community, use these preventative strategies.

At the doctor's office:

- Ask that stethoscopes and other instruments be rubbed with alcohol to remove bacteria and other microorganisms.
- Make sure doctors and nurses wash their hands before examining you or your family members.

In the school locker room:

- Make sure any cuts remain clean and covered by fresh bandages.
- Buy your child his or her own protective sports gear and don't allow sharing.
- Stress importance of hand-washing.
- Forbid sharing of towels, lipsticks, makeup, razors, or other personal items.
- Stow a bottle of Purell in your child's gym bag and ask that it be used regularly.

At the gym:

- Before going to the gym cover open cuts or sores with bandages.
- Use your own pad or mat.
- Wash your hands with liquid soap.
- Avoid bar soaps used by others that may retain bacteria.
- Wipe off equipment and weights with an antiseptic before and after you use them.
- Wash your hands and/or shower before leaving the gym.
- Bring your own towel from home or, at the very least, never share a towel with anyone.

---

bugs. There may be other probiotics out there that fit this criteria, but I am most familiar with Dr. Ohhira's Probiotics 12 PLUS, which we discussed in Chapter 2. Dr. Ohhira and his team of researchers at Okayama University in Japan isolated a lactic acid–based bacteria known as Enterococcus faecalie TH10 from the Malaysian soy tempeh. TH10 was fermented and isolated over a five-year period, resulting in a super probiotic strain potent enough to destroy the MRSAs as, well as Salmonella, E. coli, and H. pylori. Over and over, other researchers find that taking probiotics can alleviate inflammation linked to the Superbugs (especially H. pylori) and can keep these bacteria from coming back in large numbers.

Eat a high-fiber diet. As you already know, fiber helps to keep your food moving swiftly through the GI tract as well as to feed your GI Good Guy probiotics. Broccoli is a great high-fiber Superbug fighter—research shows that an antioxidant chemical in broccoli, sulforaphane, can help the body control H. pylori. In one study, after two months of eating broccoli sprouts every day, twenty people with gastritis linked to H. pylori experienced significant relief. Other high-fiber vegetables I encourage you to enjoy: turnip greens, kale, and cauliflower.

Drink some cabbage juice. A traditional treatment for ulcers, cabbage juice supports mucus in the stomach. Like broccoli, cabbage contains sulforaphane, an antioxidant that helps fight H. pylori. In one study, drinking a liter of fresh cabbage juice per day helped heal ulcers in about ten days. If that much volume doesn't seem that appealing, have a glass of cabbage juice daily with lunch.

Cook with rhubarb. This vegetable can help alleviate intestinal bleeding linked to ulcers. A study in China of more than three hundred people with ulcers found that 90 percent of them had their bleeding stop in about three days. Rhubarb's benefit is believed to stem from its astringent flavonoids and anthraquinones. Many people don't enjoy the taste of rhubarb; if this describes you, try one teaspoon of rhubarb powder every other day for two weeks between meals, and cut back to twice a week therafter.

Avoid milk and other lactose-containing products. Even if you enjoy milk and it doesn't normally bother you, E. coli infestation can cause temporary lactose intolerance and even make other symptoms worse. For this and many other reasons, I recommend that you avoid milk and become a food sleuth. Read all food labels carefully, being on the lookout not only for milk and lactose but also for milk by-products, dry milk solids, and nonfat dry milk powder. All of these contain lactose to some degree. Many medications also contain lactose.

Exercise. Try to get moving at least five times a week by walking at least twenty to thirty minutes at a time and jumping on a mini-trampoline at least five minues per day. You might even enjoy walking, biking, swimming, dancing, or some other aerobic activity. Many of these exercises will boost your cardiovascular system. The mini-trampoline gently moves the lymphatic system, your body's natural garbage disposal. The end result is that your entire immune system will be enhanced, a helpful asset in overall health and in fighting the Superbugs.

Use spices to kill Superbugs on a daily basis. These include parsley, nutmeg, cinnamon, sage, tarragon, and oregano. Capsaicin, the spicy chemical in cayenne, has been shown to kill H. pylori, as well as slow down the inflammation caused by H. pylori infestation. Turmeric, that yellowish spice that gives curry its color, contains curcumin, an immune-enhancing antioxidant and anti-inflammatory as well. A study at the University of Illinois shows that ginger may inhibit the growth of Superbugs. Aside from helping quell nausea, ginger may keep ulcers from forming. If you dislike the taste of ginger, you can take two ginger capsules with each meal.

Look into licorice. Licorice contains flavonoids that have been shown in studies to eradicate H. pylori and even be effective against H. pylori that is resistant to antibiotics. The best form to use is deglycyrrhizinated licorice

(DGL), which causes no side effects and can be used for a prolonged period of time. In a test of more than thirty people with ulcers, more than three quarters of them significantly reduced their ulcers by taking DGL; about 40 percent of the ulcer sufferers had their ulcers completely disappear. DGL supports the stomach lining, helping to boost blood supply and production of protective mucus. Take one DGL supplement daily between meals.

Make it mastic gum. This natural substance may help eradicate H. pylori that is antibiotic resistant. Take one or two capsules of mastic gum (1,000 mg per capsule) two times daily between meals. I recommend the Allergy Research Mastica.

Drink plenty of water. As I recommend throughout the Gut Flush Plan, please drink half your body weight in ounces of water every day. Not only does this help your cells remain plump and well fortified against hidden invaders, but water ensures normal bowel and kidney function to rid the body of wastes as well as stored fat. Adequate amounts of water will assist the kidneys in filtering their own waste products so the liver can begin to metabolize its own waste products without having to do the kidneys' work.

Eliminate irritating beverages. Cut out coffee and regular tea, soft drinks, and other caffeinated drinks that can aggravate your ulcer. The herbal teas that are mentioned in the 21-day plan will soothe and sustain your system.

Quiet and soothe your belly with aloe vera. Aloe vera has both antifungal and antibacterial properties. Used to treat sores and lesions since biblical times, aloe vera juice contains flavonoids that help the body heal; it binds to growth factors and speeds repair of damaged tissue. Drink two ounces of aloe vera juice daily with a meal.

Now let's turn our attention to Colon Corruptor #4, one of the most common and insidious sources of Gut Grief: food sensitivities. We might go years, or even decades, without realizing that we suffer from a food sensitivity. But when you follow the Gut Flush Plan, you'll eliminate many of the most common problem foods—and that one step may resolve many of your Gut Grief problems right off the bat.

Colon Corruptor #4: Food Sensitivities

Hannah's life was spent in a constant whirlwind of activity, although she was clearly tired and even exhausted most of the time.

She was like a "white" tornado, overcompensating for her lack of energy by pushing herself. She rushed to work. She rushed to finish her work assignments. She rushed through workouts at the gym, rushed home, and stood impatiently in her kitchen, mentally rushing her microwave to finish "cooking" her frozen dinner. She barely had time to eat before she sat down to finish more "rush" work that she had brought home from the office that she grudgingly needed to complete.

Hannah, the editor of a woman's magazine, had come to me for help because she had just reviewed an article for her magazine that linked a variety of seemingly unrelated physical and emotional symptoms with food intolerances. Hannah was having trouble focusing on her writing assignments. She suffered from frequently increasing headaches and canker sores. Her latest blood test revealed severe iron deficiency, which made her even more concerned.

To make matters worse, even though she worked out at the gym five days a week, her weight was gradually climbing. The extra pounds made Hannah feel sluggish and slow.

When we began our work together, I had Hannah keep a food diary of a typical week's worth of meals, including a weekend. She brought her diary to our next meeting, and I immediately spotted several red flags.

First of all, Hannah was an emotional eater and used food as comfort against daily stressors. She was hooked on pita chips and craved whole-grain breads and crackers with meals and as snacks.

Also—and this was a biggie—she was Italian: pasta was a basic mainstay of her diet and holiday celebrations with her large family.

Hannah knew something had to change. As gently as I could, I explained to her that many times delayed food sensitivities happen because of commonly eaten foods we eat every day. Unlike true allergies, which produce immediate histamine responses with itching or hives, a delayed food response can present itself in a variety of unsuspecting ways from two hours to two days after consumption of the troublesome food. Unresolved headaches, canker sores, and anemia are classic symptoms of gluten intolerance of one degree or another.

When I had Hannah avoid products containing gluten, including wheat, and replace them with gluten-free grains and starchy vegetables, she started losing weight on the first day of the program, without paying attention to calories, fat grams, or carb grams. After three days, her energy was better. Within a week, Hannah was no longer complaining of headaches or canker sores. It took a while for the anemia to resolve itself, but once her intestinal tract became less inflamed she was able to absorb more vitamins and minerals, including iron. All this was quite a feat for somebody who grew up on Italian food.

At first, she sheepishly admitted, her cravings for pasta almost did her in. But within a couple of days she found time to go shopping at a health food supermarket and located the rice and whole soybean pasta alternatives that I mentioned to her—and she loved them. For Hannah, following the Gut Flush Plan and getting off wheat was a lifesaver. Addressing this particular Colon Corruptor was so helpful to her that she swears she's never going back.

The three previous Colon Corruptors we talked about were obvious enemies. The very thought of yeast, parasites, and Superbugs makes us so uncomfortable that we can't seem to get rid of them fast enough. But the fourth Colon Corruptor is a tricky one, a foe that can masquerade as a friend.

A secret epidemic of hidden food sensitivities—including the gluten intolerance—has left many of us miserable and may explain some of the most tenacious symptoms of Gut Grief. This complicated issue has tormented many clients over the years, people who can't figure out why they have headaches, stomachaches, fatigue, low blood cholesterol, low blood levels of vitamins D and K, zinc, and various other nutrients, dermatitis, and various types of abdominal pain. All manner of Gut Grief mysteriously plagues their daily lives with no obvious cause.

Food sensitivities are difficult to discern for several reasons. First of all, you may be sensitive to a wide variety of foods, so you just can't eliminate one food and expect your problems to vanish. Second, many individuals don't have problems that show up right away, as explained above. Delayed food responses can manifest up to two days after the "toxic" food was ingested, so many would never suspect their symptoms were tied to food. Therefore we have to do some detective work to find the guilty items.

Luckily, in the hunt for allergies, we can point to some of the usual suspects. Unluckily, those particular suspects are often hidden in a wide variety of foods. That's why I've designed the Gut Flush Plan to help you automatically avoid the most common villains.

Let's start by taking a look at how our Food Fright environment has made allergies such a widespread problem to begin with. Then we can better understand how to Flush food sensitivities out and keep them from ruining our health.

Sense and Sensitivities

Food allergies can be scary. If you are allergic to peanuts, for example, eating a peanut or peanut butter will cause an immediate, obvious reaction—wheezing, hives, or digestive upset—that points directly to the source. About 11 million Americans have these kinds of food allergies, including 6 percent of children under age three and 3 to 4 percent of adults. Each year about thirty thousand people receive lifesaving treatment in emergency rooms after suffering severe allergic reactions to food.

While these statistics are troubling, I believe (and I'm not alone) that our adverse reactions to specific foods are as dangerous as the prevalence of acute food allergies. In her must-read book *Going Against the Grain,* my good friend Melissa Diane Smith identified delayed food responses as being more subtle and taking longer to show up than the generally recognized allergies. These can also lead to complications like food cravings, food addictions, bingeing, increased appetite, and a decreased metabolism that are not obviously the result of just an allergy.

While digestive challenges like irritable bowel syndrome (IBS) as well as heartburn/GERD, constipation, and diarrhea have all been linked with food sensitivities, there is a whole array of baffling symptoms that can spread far beyond just the digestive tract:

- unexplained mood swings and mental problems, such as panic attacks, attention deficit disorder, depression, irritability, and nervousness
- persistent pain, such as headaches, joint pain, muscle aches, arthritis
- mucus problems, such as congested nose and sinuses, runny nose, persistent phlegm, constant sneezing
- puffy eyes, dark bags, and swelling beneath the eyes
- weight that yo-yos up and down every day by as much as five pounds; edema
- chronic fatigue and extreme tiredness after eating
- Ménière's disease, an inner ear problem causing tinnitus and vertigo

You may suspect you are sensitive to certain foods and shy away from them naturally, saying things like, "Shrimp just don't seem to *agree* with me." But shrimp may just be one of many. If you suffer from unexplained symptoms of Gut Grief, you owe it to yourself to find out for sure (see Resources for food allergy testing labs).

Risk Factors for Food Sensitivities

Ninety percent of food allergies and sensitivities stem from the most common reaction-producing foods: wheat, milk, corn, unfermented soy, and peanuts. In some cases, like peanuts for example, a true allergy can lead to anaphylactic shock, a deadly allergic response in which the body releases histamines, causing tissues to swell, inhibiting breathing and interfering with blood flow, and sometimes leading to heart failure.

Make no mistake, allergies can be fatal.

Delayed "food sensitivities" are especially problematic because most health practitioners are not aware enough to recognize them. So, let's you and I take a look at some of the most common underlying factors that promote food sensitivity issues.

Antibiotics. The familiar double-edged sword we discussed previously, the overuse of antibiotics and their attack on our GI Good Guy probiotic bacteria, adds to our challenging "full-blown" allergy situation. Since probiotics in the gut moderate our immune responses, it only makes sense that they do the same for allergic reactions, restraining the overreacting inflammations of the immune system. In a study of thirty thousand children in England, scientists found that those who were given antibiotics before age one were the most likely to have hay fever, eczema, and asthma. The more medicine they were given, the more likely they were to have these allergy-related problems, another keen example that shows us why antibiotics should be avoided, if at all possible.

Too much of a few foods. The more we eat of a potentially reactive food, the greater the likelihood we are to become sensitive to that food because of constant reactions that eventually break down the immune system. That's another reason that I find today's typical diet so disturbing. As food companies and big agribusiness increase profits by increasing efficiencies of scale, they create food out of a limited palate of raw materials. If you add up all the foods that are currently made from corn, wheat, and dairy, you'll have just about all the foods at your local supermarket. Even processed food's main sweetener, high fructose corn syrup, is made from corn. Throw in a little vegetable oil to make the food less dry-tasting, and the result is that we're eating the same basic stuff, over and over and over again.

Lactose, casein, and various chemical intolerances. Lactose or milk sugar intolerance is the most common food intolerance and one of the most frequently bemoaned sources of Gut Grief. This condition affects one in ten Americans whose bodies can't make lactase, the enzyme that breaks down the lactose in milk. Another prevalent food intolerance is linked to the protein casein, which is found in milk and all cheese products. Food additives like preservatives or colors can irritate digestion and cause symptoms. Monosodium glutamate, which is used to make flavors more intense, can

CELIAC DISEASE, THE NEWLY EMERGING EPIDEMIC

■

In September 2007, *Newsweek* magazine featured an article titled "Waiter, Please Hold the Wheat," which revealed that one in 133 Americans have some form of celiac disease. As the article pointed out, celiac is becoming much more common in this country, although it is still very much underdiagnosed.

Celiac can be a difficult disease to diagnose because its random symptoms don't always point to intestinal tract. These symptoms can include anemia, osteoporosis, short stature, depression—or, possibly, no symptoms at all. This is dangerous because celiac is serious and can kill.

Celiac disease is a devastating autoimmune reaction that occurs when the presence of gluten in the small intestine causes the body to attack, and effectively destroy, the walls of the gastrointestinal tract. Celiac sufferers are unable to absorb nutrients and lose large amounts of weight; they can also endure severe pain, implacable diarrhea, bloat, and stools filled with fatty material.

Celiac can lead to microscopic colitis, IBS, even stomach and duodenal ulcers; it can make us prone to just about every autoimmune disease, such as:

- Type 1 diabetes
- Liver autoimmune disease
- Thyroid autoimmune disease (such as Hashimoto's disease, Graves' disease)
- Dermatitis herpetiformis (an intense itching of the skin)
- Autoimmune-related autism

Your diet plays an enormous role in your risk of developing, or avoiding, these conditions. An increased risk of various cancers, including cancer of the small intestine and esophagus, can just about disappear when sufferers follow a gluten-free diet. Older women with celiac are much more likely to have osteoporosis, but following a gluten-free diet can help strengthen the skeleton.

Perhaps the most frightening fact about celiac disease is that you really can have it without feeling or displaying any symptoms, while your disease silently destroys your small intestine. Research from the Mayo Clinic found that nine out of ten people with celiac don't know they have it because their symptoms are

(continued)

not obviously tied to gluten. In one study, scientists found that a group of thirty-five people with celiac had suffered with the disease for an average of twenty-eight years before doctors identified the source of difficulties. Almost three decades! If a family member has been diagnosed with celiac, or you suspect you may be at risk, don't wait another minute. Get tested!

cause severe headaches and joint pain in people who are sensitive to it. Monosodium glutamate is a type of excitotoxin, a substance that binds to brain receptors and may kill brain cells. Salicylates, chemicals related to aspirin that are in some fruits and vegetables as well as coffee, beer, and wine, have been linked to hyperactivity in children. Sulfites, which occur naturally, as in red wines, or may be added to foods to prevent the growth of mold, can also cause severe headaches.

Sensitivity to gluten. Many of my clients over the years have shown delayed food responses to grains. The chief villain is wheat, which seems to go hand in hand with fatigue, bloating, and abdominal cramping, among many other symptoms noted earlier. Aside from its starchy carbohydrates, another reason wheat causes so much Gut Grief and other problems is gluten, a sticky class of proteins also contained in barley, rye, kamut, spelt, and triticale. Gluten is widely used in processed foods because of its stickiness and ability to hold foods together.

What may be a handy binding agent for food manufacturers can also be a Colon Corruptor in our bodies. In my own practice, I have seen how gluten sensitivity leads to nutrient malabsorption as well as leaky gut syndrome. As the intestinal villi are harmed and atrophy, the whole process of taking in crucial nutrients goes haywire. In addition, larger molecules like protein fragments breach the damaged GI walls, enter the bloodstream, and cause widespread allergic reactions. As those proteins circulate in the body, they activate the immune system, causing inflammation and triggering certain devastating autoimmune diseases. All this destruction is created by a condition that can be avoided by simply choosing different foods. But awareness is the biggest hurdle.

YOUR BRAIN ON GLUTEN

■

The part of your body most sensitive to gluten might not be your gut but your head. Those with celiac are prone to polyneuropathy, a condition that damages peripheral nerves and can lead to persistent pain, weakness, trouble keeping your balance, and numbness. Research into celiac shows that it's possible that more than half of all people who have unexplained neurological malfunction of this sort may have gluten sensitivity.

Celiac can also muddle your thought processes. A study at the Mayo Clinic found that when celiac patients who were suffering cognitive decline were put on a gluten-free diet, their mental capacities improved or were at least stabilized.

The mechanism with which gluten sensitivity affects the brain and nerves hasn't been identified. The Mayo Clinic researchers think nerve damage may occur because of nutrient deficiencies linked to celiac, like a lack of B vitamins, or the cause may be inflammation brought on by autoimmune attacks on brain tissue. But they stress that you improve the most if you go off gluten at the earliest possible moment and not wait until nerve and brain problems are firmly entrenched.

Along with many of my colleagues, I have noted that the issue of gluten sensitivity resembles a giant iceberg. At the visible tip are those who know they have celiac disease—these people have given up gluten because they suffered so much when they ate wheat and other gluten-containing foods. Beneath the surface are people who have a silent version of this problem and don't know it yet (see "Celiac Disease, the Newly Emerging Epidemic," page 79). And perhaps the largest group below the water line is made up of those who suffer milder gluten sensitivity symptoms but don't experience full-blown celiac disease.

Still don't think it could be you? Upward of 70 percent of us have inherited a genetic tendency for gluten sensitivity, and experts estimate about half of the general population has some degree of it. And while it takes, on average, about eleven years for someone with celiac disease to be diagnosed, those who are gluten sensitive may never realize that their health problems are linked to a gluten reaction.

Let's try to make sure that you're not one of them.

Do You Have a Food Sensitivity?

Even if you don't think you have a food sensitivity, take a moment to complete the following questionnaire—you may be surprised. Your answers can indicate the probability that you suffer from food sensitivities.

Are you often clumsy and uncoordinated?
Do you have itchy skin, chronic skin rashes, or eczema?
Do you suffer unexplained headaches?
Do you have irritable bowel syndrome?
Do you eat the same foods day after day?
Are you frequently the victim of food cravings?
Are you a compulsive eater?
Has your metabolism slowed down?
Do you suffer from a lot of water retention?
Do you engage in binge eating?
Do you sometimes suffer from nausea, confusion, and agitation?

Are you often subject to abdominal cramping?

Do you have breathing problems, like wheezing?

Do you frequently sneeze?

Do you often feel bloated?

Are you often depressed for no reason?

Have you been diagnosed with early-onset osteoporosis, and do you take
enough calcium, magnesium, and vitamin D?

If you answered yes to any of these questions, you may be suffering from a food sensitivity. If you suspect you have a full-blown allergy or celiac disease, ask your doctor if you're a candidate for a blood test (see Resources).

The Gut Flush Food Sensitivity Protocol

For most of us, sensitivities seem to cluster around a few ordinary foods, mostly wheat, corn, and milk. Interestingly, there may also be herbs and spices that you have a reaction to and are simply not aware of. For example, black pepper is a frequent culprit. If your results from the survey above suggest that food sensitivities are derailing your health, try the following suggestions to help tip the balance in your favor.

Learn to speak the lingo. If you suspect you're sensitive to ingredients like MSG, learn about its alternate names on labels. On packaging, MSG may be referred to as hydrolyzed soy protein, autolyzed plant protein, or hydrolyzed vegetable protein. Unfortunately, MSG may even be something as seemingly innocuous as "natural flavorings."

Practice an elimination diet. When you think you are gluten-intolerant or sensitive to a particular food, try an elimination diet to help you identify the problem more precisely. Consult the "The Top Three Food Sensitivities" chart (page 84) to consider some common sources of food sensitivities, and then follow this process to systematically narrow down your list of suspects.

- Choose a food that you routinely eat and eliminate it first.
- Cut out all dishes made with this item from your meals at home.
- When shopping, read labels to see if any undesirable ingredient is listed.

- In restaurants, always consult with your server about the preparation of your food. You can't always tell from the menu exactly what's in a dish. Explain your problem and the restaurant should accommodate your special needs.
- Continue to avoid the suspected food for two to three weeks, keeping a simple log to help you notice if your symptoms ease.
- If symptoms disappear, briefly reintroduce the food and see if they return.
- If they do, you know you need to permanently drop that food from your diet.

THE TOP THREE FOOD SENSITIVITIES

Foods with Gluten: Wheat bran, wheat germ, cracked wheat, einkorn, emmer, spelt, kamut, wheat starch, hydrolyzed wheat protein, rye, barley, triticale, and all baked goods; candies, modified food starch, processed meats, crumb toppings, thickeners, ale, beer, Postum, many flours (bromated, durum, enriched, graham, phosphated, plain, self-rising, white, semolina), farina, bouillon cubes; cold cuts, including hot dogs, salami, sausage; wafers, gravy, fake fish (imitation), matzo, self-basting turkeys, pita chips, soy sauce.

Foods with Corn: High fructose corn syrup, fructose, cornstarch, corn flour, tortillas, tacos, corn chips, corn oil, cornmeal, corn cereals, baking powder, popcorn, hominy grits, cranberry juice and other juices and fruit drinks, corn bread, hydrolyzed vegetable protein, wax on fresh fruit, margarine, hot dogs and sausage, salad dressings, mayonnaise, baby foods, breaded frozen fish, cough drops, chewing gum, soft drinks, crackers, bread, buns, rolls, whiskey, energy bars, candy bars.

Foods with Milk and Casein Products: Whole milk, skim, 1 percent, and 2 percent milk; chocolate milk, flavored milks, buttermilk, sour cream, ice cream, cream cheese, ricotta, mozzarella, cottage cheese, cheddar cheese, American cheese, feta cheese, cheese spreads and processed cheese, all hard and aged cheeses, pizza, condensed milk, butter, ghee, whey, chocolate (and other candy) bars, energy bars, custard, nougat, rice (and other) puddings, half-and-half, lactose.

GLUTEN-FREE FOODS

Amaranth	Legumes	Seeds
Arrowroot	Millet	Soy
Buckwheat	Nuts	Sorghum
Cassava	Quinoa	Tapioca
Flax	Rice	Wild Rice
Indian rice grass	Sago	Yucca
Job's tears		

Focus on "safe" foods. Enough of my clients have shown risk factors for gluten sensitivity that when I see the first blush of symptoms, I usually recommend they eliminate gluten from their diets. To be honest, aside from a bit of a learning curve, there is truly no nutritional downside. In this case, consider eliminating all of the foods in the gluten section of the "The Top Three Food Sensitivities" chart and substitute the foods in the "Gluten-free Foods" list (above). The upside is, even if you don't have a bona fide gluten sensitivity, you'll automatically be eating fewer corrosive carbohydrates, which can only help you Fortify and Flush your gut even faster. The Gut Flush eating and supplement plan, which begins on page 87, does this automatically for you.

Ease food sensitivities by easing stress. Studies have shown that exercise and other stress-reducers can help alleviate or moderate allergies. Try a few of these strategies to immediately help manage fallout from your food sensitivities.

- *Walk daily.* Thirty minutes of walking a day can reduce stress, tone your immune system, and reduce your risk of allergies.
- *Have a massage once a week.* The easy, rhythmic experience of a massage can help improve blood circulation and ease anxiety.
- *Take a yoga class twice a week.* Ask your instructor for particular yoga postures that can boost circulation, tone muscles, and ease health problems linked to excess stress.

- *Focus on your breathing.* Research on meditation shows that easy, controlled breathing may help the body deal with allergies. First thing in the morning, don't just pop out of bed—slowly breathe in and out, focusing on the movements of your diaphragm. Spend three to five minutes consciously relaxing and breathing.

Take fish oil on a daily basis. Fish oil is a natural anti-inflammatory and may modulate allergy-type symptoms. The essential fatty acids in fish oil play a key role in cardiovascular, brain, joint, and immune system health.

Continue to fit in your Gut Flush Basic Protocol probiotics. Help your probiotic population boost your body's immune system response and put a damper on inflammation triggered by food sensitivities by staying current with your Gut Flush Basic Protocol. Also, be sure to eat your probiotic foods daily, such as a cup of yogurt.

Allow antioxidants to do their work. Antioxidants help the body cope with any aftereffects of allergic reactions and fight oxidative stress. I recommend Oxi-Key from Uni Key (see Resources), which contains catalase, superoxide dismutase, glutathione, N-acetylcysteine, L-cysteine, vitamin B_2, vitamin E, and thioproline.

We've come to the most exciting part of the program, the core of the Gut Flush Plan. I've taken special care to design this three-stage eating and supplement plan to help *anyone*—no matter their age, physical condition, or sex—achieve optimum digestive health.

In the next chapter, we'll begin with the first stage: Fortify. You'll learn how to strengthen your digestive system's natural defenses by using specific foods that help your GI Good Guys thrive. By improving your "terrain," you will reduce your risk of falling victim to the next Food Fright disaster.

The three-stage Gut Flush Plan really opens the door to enhanced immunity, soaring personal energy, trouble-free digestion, and total health. I'm excited to share it with you.

Let's begin.

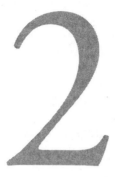

How the Gut Flush Plan Works

7

Step 1: Fortify

IF YOU'VE BEGUN TO USE YOUR GUT FLUSH BASIC PROTOCOL, YOU MAY already be feeling some of the health benefits—maybe your diarrhea or constipation has cleared up, or your skin seems smoother, or you feel more focused and clear.

After learning about the four fearsome Colon Corruptors—yeast, parasites, Superbugs, and food sensitivities—perhaps you were able to home in on a particular issue and have started one of those protocols as well.

Congratulations—you're well on your way to a greater sense of vitality and sparkling health!

Now it's time to take it to the next level, to incorporate a holistic nutritional approach that will help you feel lighter, more energetic, blissfully safe, and free from all sorts of food-borne illnesses—no matter what your particular circumstances may be.

In the next three chapters you'll learn all the specifics of how the Gut Flush Plan can Fortify, Flush, and Feed that precious digestive tract of yours. If you're currently following one of the protocols for a Colon Corruptor, by all means continue. If you're lucky enough to be starting the Gut Flush Plan without a Colon Corruptor, so much the better. The Gut Flush Plan is designed to work with each of those protocols or all by itself.

For the first stage of the core Gut Flush eating and supplement plan, we'll focus on Fortifying your digestive tract. Let's consider why Fortifying is our primary objective on the plan.

Terrain Is Everything

As the story goes, the great researcher and scientist Louis Pasteur had a long-standing argument with scientist Antoine Bechamp. Pasteur, the creator of the germ theory, believed that most health problems were the result of germs. Bechamp, on the other hand, thought an unhealthy inner terrain or ecology gave rise to the germs.

On his deathbed, Pasteur relented and finally acknowledged that Bechamp was correct: the microbe is nothing; the terrain is everything.

I couldn't agree more.

Most of us don't get sick just because we have the unfortunate luck of picking up a bug. We are more likely the victim of toxic overload because we are harboring an internal environment—a type of terrain—that makes the body hospitable to pathogens like yeast, fungus, parasites, worms, and undesirable Superbugs.

On the other hand, when the intestinal tract's terrain is in balance, with enough probiotic bacteria and the proper interior acidic environment, harmful microorganisms are crowded out with no available place to cause trouble. Pathogens may come and go, but thanks to the natural cooperation between your immune system and probiotics, you remain healthy.

This kind of "bulletproof" terrain is the first objective of the Gut Flush Plan. Once your terrain is Fortified and strong enough to deflect any new invaders, your gut can concentrate its resources on Flushing out the existing ones. Then you can move on to Feeding the gut lining, ensuring strong resistance in the future, and allowing it to completely heal from any former abuse.

Let's begin the Gut Flush Plan by looking at the six most important strategies to Fortify your digestive tract's natural defenses.

Fortify Tactic #1: Single Out All Remaining Sweets, Molds, and Starches

If you've been following the protocol for any of the Colon Corruptors, you've already gone a long way in eliminating foods that encourage their activity. Now we're going to close ranks and shut down their energy sources altogether. The first tactic of Fortify is to target any lingering foods and beverages that are contraindicated for *any* of the underlying parasites, yeast, Superbugs, or hidden food sensitivities. And that means tossing the remaining sweets, molds, and starches.

Let's not beat around the bush: when it comes to overall health, sugar is dietary enemy No. 1. And sugar's kissin' cousin, the artificial sweetener, also does you no favors. That's why, for the initial two weeks of the 21-Day Gut Flush Plan, you will not use sugar or artificial sweeteners in any form. That means no fruits, fruit juice, sugar alcohols (including xylitol), or even natural sweeteners like honey, maple syrup, or agave. (One exception: As you will note in the menu plans, you can use the powdered Flora-Key [see Resources] as your Gut Flush sugar substitute, thanks to a special ingredient in this product that acts as a natural sweetener and prebiotic. We'll talk more about why prebiotics are so important in Fortify Tactic #2.)

In my experience, sugar, natural sweeteners, and artificial sweeteners feed parasites and yeast and/or create bloating in the gut, making us feel (and, unfortunately, look) fatter. This bloating occurs because many of our guts have become so dysfunctional that we have trouble absorbing these nutrients. We also have trouble absorbing any of the sweeteners, no matter what kind they are. Some studies show that a staggering nine out of ten of us bloat and have trouble digesting our food when we eat sweeteners.

When you eat sugar and other highly refined starchy carbs (such as white bread, white rice, white pasta), or even too many grains and naturally starchy vegetables, the Colon Corruptors in your gut rejoice—and quickly begin a feeding frenzy. Bacteria and yeast seize upon these foods and easily ferment them, releasing detrimental enzymes that ravenously feast on the sugar you eat. This process discharges large amounts of gas that swell your digestive tract and give you that uncomfortable bloated feeling, which in some very severe cases, can push up your stomach, making you feel as if you are having a heart attack.

Just picture the bubbles fizzing and popping in a glass of champagne—that's actually what's happening inside you when those microorganisms set to work. Scientific tests show that when a person experiences bloat, their breath has traces of alcohol in it. And just like that bottle of champagne, you can feel like you're about to pop.

In addition to feeding yeast, many sugary foods may already have yeast in them, and by eating yeast-containing foods, you introduce even more yeast cells into your intestines. If your digestion is not up to the job of completely absorbing carbohydrates, when these foods get farther along in the intestines, instead of being absorbed, they just provide even more company for already existing yeast.

Colon Corruptors thrive on foods that contain yeast and mold, such as cheese, mushrooms, vinegars (with the exception of apple cider vinegar), soy sauce, tamari, wine, beer, and vitamins that are yeast derived. The 21-Day Gut Flush Plan menus and recipes specifically avoid these foods for that very reason.

We know starchy foods feed Colon Corruptors just as readily as sugar does, so we'll certainly want to toss any foods containing gluten or corn—both also major sources of food sensitivity (as discussed in Chapter 6). Instead of foods that contain wheat, rye, barley, or corn, you'll be enjoying hearty, delicious Fortifying dinners that will delight your taste buds with brown rice, quinoa, and amaranth.

Now that we've cut off the Colon Corruptors' supply lines, let's help support the troops that fight them—probiotics.

Fortify Tactic #2: Power Up on Probiotics and Prebiotics

By now you know what incredible foot soldiers probiotics are in the war against Colon Corruptors. The original GI Good Guys, probiotics help keep the peace and make sure to keep your gut's health balance tipped in your favor. In addition to crowding out Colon Corruptors, in a beneficial way they also ferment the fiber that our digestive tracts can't break down and help create an acidic environment that keeps the GI tract healthy. We depend on probiotics to keep the digestive process functioning, so we have to make sure we support them.

I hope you've already begun to incorporate probiotics into your daily routine with the Gut Flush Basic Protocol. Now it's time to call in more reinforcements.

Add One Probiotic Food Daily

In the Gut Flush Plan, you'll include at least *one* probiotic food (such as one cup of plain yogurt or kefir, a half cup of sauerkraut, or one cup of plain miso) every day.

Many people are surprised when I tell them that sauerkraut and pickles help them protect their probiotic population—they think these foods' acidic nature "kills" the GI Good Guys. But, actually, humans have used the bacteria in these fermented foods to protect their health and bolster food preservation for millennia.

Traditional fermentation is based on a pretty simple principle. The process allows particular airborne bacteria to grow in food and keep it from spoiling. These bacteria—known as lactic acid bacteria—not only keep food edible but also offer remarkable therapeutic advantages when you swallow them. In your body, these organic acids keep the bowels from becoming too alkaline. Without this acidity, the beneficial flora in the colon wilt and start to die off.

As long ago as 1908, the Russian scientist Dr. Elie Metchnikoff, who received a Nobel Prize for his work on probiotics in the twentieth century, pointed out that undesirable bacteria living in the gut could produce a toxic inner environment that wreaks havoc on health and gives rise to life-threatening conditions. He discovered that beneficial bacteria in fermented foods (he focused on those in yogurt) could crowd out pathogens and boost health. It wasn't until almost one hundred years later that mainstream medical researchers caught up with Dr. Metchnikoff's ideas and proved him right. In fact, many experts credit good gut flora with several amazing actions. They believe probiotics:

- prevent all kinds of different diseases, especially chronic degenerative ones;

- help control inflammation, a central feature of so many degenerative diseases including heart disease;
- increase antibodies to fight off infections;
- improve digestion;
- have anticancer properties.

Consider this real-life story told in the October 2004 issue of the *Women's Health Newsletter* by my colleague Nan Fuchs, Ph.D. It shows how the right kind of probiotic can even save your life.

The doctor told Joan that her ninety-five-year-old mother, Bernice, was unlikely to survive the night. The massive doses of antibiotics she had been given for her severe bacterial infection were not working. Her doctor advised against giving her any probiotics because he didn't know what they were.

But Joan felt there was nothing to lose. She knew that probiotics were beneficial bacteria that fight harmful ones, so she gave Bernice the strongest probiotic formula I'd ever found. The next morning her mother was sitting up in bed and eating!

"I saw a tunnel," she told Joan. "At the end was a white light and lots and lots of white clouds." She had also seen her parents and long-dead husband. Bernice had certainly been close to death. Now she was back for a while, thanks to a probiotic (Dr. Ohhira's Probiotics 12 PLUS to be exact) so strong it's been shown in university-based studies to kill antibiotic-resistant Superbugs.

Don't expect results like this from just any probiotic supplement. Many have very little activity; they may help your digestion or reduce your Candida symptoms, but they won't turn your health around the way the best formulas can. Unfortunately, you can't judge probiotics by the company that sells them. Some good supplement companies sell friendly bacteria that don't do much (see "Pick the Right Probiotic," page 95, for more information on how to select the best brands).

Add Two Prebiotics Daily

Because probiotics are living organisms, we'll need to keep them well fed. To that end, we'll also add two daily servings of foods such as onions, garlic, oregano, Jerusalem artichokes, leeks, and jicama, all types of *prebiotics,* the main food source of probiotics in the body.

PICK THE RIGHT PROBIOTIC

You can get millions of CFUs (colony-forming units) in probiotic foods, but certain probiotic supplements provide CFUs in the billions, providing more potent therapeutic benefits. Use the following criteria to select the highest-quality probiotic supplement. Your probiotic should:

- have living bacteria that ensures the bacteria are alive and active;
- be packaged in a fermented culture, which contains the nutrients in which the beneficial lactic acid bacteria have been nurtured and developed with their own continual feeding system;
- include organic acids, which the bacteria utilize to keep the colon's pH acidic level high enough to further promote the growth of good bacteria;
- be enteric coated to keep it intact and able to survive harsh stomach and bile acids after you swallow it until it travels to the colon;
- provide evidence that the benefits of the supplement have been confirmed by third-party research and that it is gluten free, non-GMO, hypoallergenic, with no preservatives;
- have proven adhesion: that means it sticks to the walls of the digestive tract and therefore is 100 percent effective;
- be safe for infants, children, women, and men, as well as individuals with a compromised immune system;
- have multiple strains of beneficial bacteria that have been confirmed by research:

  Bifidobacterium breve ss. Breve

  Bifidobacterium infantis ss. Infantis

  Bifidobacterium longum

  Lactobacillus brevis

  Lactobacillus acidophilus

  Lactobacillus bulgaricus

  Lactobacillus casei ss. Casei

  Lactobacillus fermentum

  Lactobacillus helveticus ss. Jagurti

(continued)

Prebiotics are a type of nondigestible sugar molecule that feeds the good bacteria without nurturing the bad. The most well known prebiotic is one called fructooligosaccharides, or FOS, from fruits and vegetables. Another prebiotic is inulin. Both feed the friendly bifidobacteria in the large intestine. Inulin is specifically used to increase fiber and reduce fats and sugars.

Foods like chicory root, asparagus, and shallots offer up high levels of inulin. The Gut Flush Plan will add two prebiotic foods to your diet every day, to help Feed your good bacteria and Fortify your gut.

STRONG PROBIOTICS EQUAL STRONG BONES

Healthy probiotics in the gut protect the whole body. That includes even your bones. Research now shows that osteoporosis can be connected to a lack of probiotic bacteria in your colon. Scientists at Baylor University found that probiotics boost calcium absorption. When adolescents were given prebiotic supplements, the fiber that feeds probiotics, their calcium absorption rose dramatically—by an extra 11 grams annually.

Other research shows that the acidic environment created in the colon by probiotics and fermented foods plays a big role in calcium assimilation. Without an acidic colon, calcium absorption slips and your chances for both osteoporosis and colon cancer, linked to poor calcium metabolism, may subsequently rise. When you bolster your probiotic population, you are also boning up on calcium.

Fortify Tactic #3: Fill Up on Soluble Fiber

You've heard many medical experts trumpet the importance of eating fiber. They'll probably tell you that fiber is supposed to keep you regular, forming the bulk that helps keep your bowel movements from being difficult. While I'm not arguing that that feature is important, the real advantage of fiber is how it helps probiotic bacteria to thrive.

All fiber is divided into two kinds—soluble and insoluble. Insoluble fiber does not dissolve in water. Forming what is known as roughage, insoluble fiber helps add bulk to your stool and helps prevent constipation. You find insoluble fiber in such foods as bran, whole grains, and nuts.

Soluble fiber, on the other hand, does dissolve in water. It can be found in green beans and dark green leafy vegetables, the skins of fruits and root vegetables, and seeds. In the digestive tract, it joins up with water to form a gooey gel. Among its other benefits, that gel helps moderate the absorption of sugars from the digestive tract into the bloodstream and balances rises in blood sugar. That, and the fact that it provides a feeling of fullness, can help control your appetite.

Most important, though, soluble fiber is also a prebiotic that nurtures probiotics. When you consume soluble fiber, you give your probiotics food they use to grow on. As probiotics ferment this fiber, they also form what are called short-chain fatty acids. Among their many benefits, these acids wield the chemical warfare that limits bad bugs like E. coli. These natural substances also inhibit the growth of Candida, holding it in check while helping heal the digestive tract.

While providing nutrients to the wall of the colon, short-chain fatty acids also tamp down inflammation. When inflammation becomes chronic and continues unabated, it can contribute to asthma, rheumatoid arthritis, inflammatory bowel disease, psoriasis, multiple sclerosis, Alzheimer's, type 2 diabetes, and cancer. In some way that researchers don't entirely understand, the presence of short-chain fatty acids convinces immune cells to stand down and call off inflammatory processes in the colon. These short-chain fatty acids, especially butyric acid, which can be found in the product ButyrEn by Allergy Research, also stimulate other immune cells that travel around the body so that they signal a general end to inflammation. That's a big benefit, and one the Gut Flush Plan ensures you will benefit from.

On a daily basis, the Gut Flush Plan includes at least *two* food sources that are rich in soluble fiber, such as oatmeal, vegetables, seeds, and nuts, and at least *one to two tablespoons* of ground flaxseed. (For those with a sensitive digestion, please grind your nuts and seeds to a fine powder.) Since it is nearly impossible to consume a diet containing the recommended 25–35 grams of daily fiber, you may wish to supplement with fiber-rich formulas that contain a blend of soluble and insoluble fiber, such as the Super-GI Cleanse (see Resources) or Inuflora and Fiber Delights (both available at health food stores).

Fortify Tactic #4: Omega-size!

You may have heard the news about fish oil helping to increase heart health and protect against arrhythmia, arterial plaque, or high blood pressure. But you may not know that the omega-3 fatty acids in fish and flaxseed oil also significantly boost digestive health. These fatty acids are incorporated directly into the cell membranes, Fortifying the body and strengthening the system by making the membranes more permeable to vital nutrients.

One of the ways omega-3s reduce the risk of heart disease—by reducing damaging inflammation—has also been shown to help control the inflammatory disease ulcerative colitis. Sometimes inflammation is a perfectly healthy response—your immune cells are simply fighting off an infection. But when inflammation occurs during colitis, it inadvertently damages the lining of the intestinal tract. The immune cells needlessly attack a problem that really isn't there, and the inflammation itself becomes the problem. That's when omegas can really help. For example, one study found that among people who were taking prescription medication to control their colitis, fish oil allowed them to cut back on their pharmaceutical medicine.

And this is perhaps most impressive: even though omega-3 fats help limit damaging inflammation, they regulate it in a way that generally doesn't limit or otherwise interfere with the body's response to real pathogenic threats. Fish oil apparently decreases inflammation by altering the body's production of what are termed prostaglandins. Prostaglandins are natural chemicals the body makes from fats that influence a wide variety of functions in the human body. As well as mediating inflammation, different types of prostaglandins control cell growth, blood clotting, and the function of muscle cells. Normally, the body makes inflammatory prostaglandins from omega-6 fats, the kind of fat in soy oil and corn oil. But fish oil effectively blocks this process by joining up with the places in cells where the prostaglandin manufacture would otherwise take place.

Taking fish oil and eating cooked fish (not sushi.) can also help the body defend itself against parasitic invasion. Trichinosis, a parasite that can be ingested from undercooked pork, strikes 11 million worldwide every year. In a laboratory study of infection by trichinosis, researchers found that fish oil supplements improved the immune response against the growth of trichinella, reducing worms and larvae of trichinosis by more than 30 percent.

Simply including more omega-3s and fewer processed omega-6s in your diet can actually help improve the body's response to intestinal parasites. Plus, when researchers examined EPA and DHA (eicosapentaenoic acid and docosahexaenoic acid), the two main types of omega-3 fatty acids, they found that these two acids can kill bacteria and are effective against E. coli O157:H7 (a type of Superbug that often causes the recall of hamburger meat), Salmonella, and staph infections.

When you follow the Gut Flush Plan, you'll eat at least four ounces of omega-3-rich fatty fish (salmon, tuna, mackerel, sardines) *twice* a week. You can also enjoy omega-3-filled nuts like walnuts and Brazil nuts on salads or as snacks. You'll incorporate at least one tablespoon *each* of fish and flaxseed oil daily in nonheated recipes. (The lemon-flavored fish oil is really quite tasty, so don't be put off by the name—it is totally nonfishy.) Also, on Week One of the 21-Day Gut Flush Plan, you may enjoy up to one tablespoon of olive oil daily (high in the nonessential but healthy omega-9-rich fatty acids) in cooking.

Fortify Tactic #5: Drink to Your Health!

Keeping your body well hydrated is one of the best ways you have to Fortify yourself against pathogens and parasites. Think of all those little bugs coming down the digestive tract, just looking for a home. The right liquids keep your cells plumped up and resistant to their infection. Without adequate hydration, even the first line of your defense, your saliva (which is normally packed with enzymes and immune cells) simply dries up—and those bugs head straight into your system. To counter this risk, the Gut Flush Plan has a multifaceted approach to hydration.

Drink Half Your Body Weight in Ounces of Water Daily

Bottom line: adequate water is crucial for good health. Research shows that when you don't get enough water, you may suffer more colds and flu; when you cut yourself, you'll take longer to heal. Become dehydrated and you have a bigger chance of urinary infections, even kidney failure and seizures.

As you age, water may become even more important. If you let yourself get dehydrated, you have a greater risk of constipation, breaking bones because of falling, as well as a higher risk of bladder cancer. But lots of studies show that people just aren't getting the bare minimum recommendation of sixty-four ounces a day. When researchers examined older people who were coming into hospital emergency rooms for various reasons, they were staggered to find that the lab work on their blood showed that about half of them were dehydrated.

Part of the problem is that as you get a little older, your body doesn't rehydrate as quickly as when you're younger, even after you take in sufficient water. You also just don't feel thirsty enough to keep enough water in your system. In a study that took men ages twenty to sixty up and down hills for some heavy hiking, researchers found that the older men were less thirsty than the younger men. The result: the guys in their fifties became dehydrated while the fellows in their twenties spontaneously drank plenty of water and stayed hydrated.

All of those are great reasons to get plenty of water each day. Each day consume *at least half of your body weight in ounces* to fully hydrate your system. One caution, though—don't drink your water with meals. Save the water until you're done eating. You see, when your food enters the digestive tract, your gut secretes those miraculous digestive enzymes that act as catalysts that help break it down into its individual nutrients. But if you swallow a lot of water at the same time, these marvelous natural chemicals become diluted and don't work as efficiently. So go easy on the water you swallow with your entrée.

Drink Two Cups of Fortifying Beverages Daily

At this stage of the program, I would really like you to eliminate coffee, especially if you are a heavy-duty coffee drinker and/or constipation is an issue for you. As discussed earlier in the book, despite the widespread belief that coffee helps to maintain regularity, it is in fact a constipation culprit. Like other stimulants and addictive laxatives, coffee bypasses the regular neuromuscular network of the colon and actually contributes to the atrophy of your nerves and muscles in the colon.

During Week One, I would like you to add at least two cups per day of a Fortifying beverage such as roasted chicory root tea or a coffee substitute such as dandelion root or caffeine-free organic African honeybush tea that my readers tell me is the closest thing to coffee. Both are available in health food stores. The roasted chicory root comes in bulk and you would use about two teaspoons in a tea ball and steep in hot water. The roasted chicory root, dandelion, and African honeybush tea can be enjoyed during or after a meal. These beverages have been shown to help to Fortify the gut, as well as boost many other health benefits.

In addition to helping lower your risk of cancer, chicory root tea is rich in inulin, the prebiotic I mentioned in Fortify Tactic #3. Other studies show that chicory can lower your chances of developing intestinal problems like dysentery, which is caused by pathogenic bacteria. In one test, researchers gave chicory to a group of people and then compared the bacteria in their stool samples to those of other folks who didn't consume any. Aside from finding that the chicory helped folks go to the bathroom more often (it's a gentle laxative), they discovered that it stimulated the growth of probiotics and reduced the amount of pathogenic bacteria measured in their gut.

Dandelion root tea is a Fortifier of the liver, your most important ally in healthy detoxification and cleansing. It has been used for decades as a gentle but highly effective natural cleansing agent and is high in potassium, one of the most important minerals for nurturing the liver.

African honeybush tea is a caffeine-free beverage made from a plant that is a native of South Africa. It has a pleasing, slightly sweet taste, and when made into a tea, it gives off an aroma similar to that of honey. While tea is filled with chemicals called tannins (which give tea its distinctive astringent taste), African honeybush is lacking these chemicals. Traditionally, African honeybush has been used to soothe throats and ease problematic coughs. Laboratory tests of African honeybush show that it is rich in antioxidants called xanthone mangifern as well as hesperitin and isokuranetin. It also contains phytoestrogens, which can help ease menopausal problems.

If you're still dubious about giving up your java habit, let me share a few disturbing facts with you. In addition to the whammy it does to your digestive system, coffee has been linked to an increased risk of rheumatoid arthritis—the more coffee you drink, the bigger the danger. If you drink four or more cups daily, your risk is double that of those who drink less. If you are a complete java fanatic, drinking upward of eleven cups to keep you going every day, your risk of rheumatoid arthritis is fifteen times (yikes!) the risk of noncoffee drinkers.

Drinking lots of unfiltered coffee also raises the risk of heart disease. Research in the Netherlands found that coffee can raise your blood levels of homocysteine, a protein linked to heart problems and stroke. In addition, pregnant women who drink eight or more cups of coffee double their risk of stillbirth. And if you drink more than eight cups, the risk is tripled.

If you have a heavy coffee habit and you decide to kick it, do so consciously and cautiously—giving up coffee and the stimulant drug of caffeine can cause headaches, bad moods, trouble concentrating, fatigue, flulike sniffles, vomiting, muscle pain, and stiffness. In tests, half of the coffee addicts suffered headaches when they stayed away from the brew. The problems come on about a day or two after stopping coffee consumption, and effects can last up to nine days, if you've been mainlining coffee. When you decide to taper off, I suggest you start by reducing your coffee consumption by alternating with dandelion root tea or chicory root tea. Every day, try one cup less until you can give up coffee completely.

Fortify Tactic #6: Shake That Salt Shaker!

Salting food is believed by some to be the oldest technique for protecting food against spoiling and being infested with bacteria that can make us sick. Over the ages, this food preservative and pathogen killer has been so valuable that even ancient Roman soldiers were paid (at least partly) in salt—and that word in Latin (*sal*) is the origin of today's word "salary." In addition to just plain tasting salty and killing pathogens, salting your food actually brings out its natural flavors—that's actually the reason why people like the taste of salted food.

Few people realize how powerful an antiseptic and natural preservative salt is. Salt interferes with the reproduction of a wide variety of bacteria,

EXTRA FORTIFICATION FOR YOUR COLON: CASTOR OIL PACKS

■

Since ancient times, castor oil has been used as a healing oil for a variety of maladies but especially for those related to the liver and gallbladder. The frequent use of a castor oil pack will help to fortify both the liver and gallbladder, which are very important organs for neutralizing, eliminating, and breaking down wastes and fat-soluble toxins through the bile. Experts believe that the oil can penetrate deeply—as much as four inches—into the body.

People who use castor oil packs on a daily basis report that they experience a higher sense of well-being and energy, as well as a normalizing effect of liver enzymes. Since the emotion of anger is so closely tied to the liver, you may find that angry feelings can start to resurface. Stay with those feelings and pledge to love and respect yourself.

You will need four things that are readily available in health food stores throughout the country or from the Heritage Store online (www.caycecures .com). These items are 100 percent pure cold-pressed castor oil, wool flannel, a heating pad, and clear plastic wrap.

Here's what you do:

1. Fold the wool flannel into three or four layers and soak with castor oil.
2. Put the flannel in a baking dish and heat it slowly in the oven until it becomes hot—but not hot enough to injure your skin.
3. Rub castor oil on your abdominal area, lie down, and place the hot flannel on top of your stomach area.
4. Seal off the flannel with Saran Wrap or a similar plastic film.
5. Cover with a heating pad for an hour, keeping the flannel as hot as safely and comfortably possible.

When you finish, wash the oil from your stomach. You can keep the oil-soaked flannel sealed in Saran Wrap or place it in a Ziploc plastic bag for further use. For a gentle detox, I recommend that you use the castor oil pack once a day for three successive days, take three days off, and then use it one more time to correlate to the first week of the 21-Day Gut Flush Plan.

molds, and other pathogens by making chemical changes on their cell membranes that suck the water (and the life) out of these bugs. Researchers have proved that it kills E. coli O157:H7, one of the most dangerous problematic forms of bacteria that can cause food poisoning. Salt can also kill bacterium Listeria monocytogenes, which frequently leads to food poisoning.

The salt that is generally available today is "evaporative" salt. It is manufactured by inserting water into underground salt deposits, a procedure that forms brine as the water wears away and dissolves salt. When the brine is boiled, and the water is removed, the salt is crystallized. The resulting crystals are of varying sizes. I prefer good old-fashioned Morton's canning and pickling salt rather than sea salt (I wonder about the mercury) or kosher salt (which contains an undesirable additive).

Since salt is such a powerful antiseptic, I recommend that you aim for at least one teaspoon a day, with some salt at every meal. My only reservation would be for those with a medical condition that otherwise prohibits the use of sodium chloride, such as those people with high blood pressure, heart problems, or ulcer difficulties. For example, salt can induce genetic changes in H. pylori, causing the bug and any resulting ulcer to grow even more virulent.

In addition, if you are African-American and have a tendency toward high blood pressure, you should go easy on the salt. Researchers find that African-Americans are more sensitive to salt than Caucasians and suffer more hypertension when under stress and eating a high-salt diet. But with those caveats in mind, salt on your food makes an excellent antimicrobial additive.

We're now ready to move on to Week Two of the Gut Flush Plan: Flush. This topic is near and dear to my heart, since I have been on the warpath against yeast, parasites, Superbugs, and food intolerances for decades. Now you can fight all of these Colon Corruptors all at once with a foolproof diet plan.

8

Step 2: Flush

Now that you've learned how to Fortify your system against any new incoming invaders, you have also given your body a boost to prepare it for Step 2. Good for you. Now let's move on to the next stage of your clean sweep. Our intent for Week Two is to really concentrate on flushing out parasites and yeast. We also want to continue to sidestep the most common food sensitivities, to make your internal ecology as unfriendly as possible to any and all Superbugs.

In the previous chapters, we've already begun to cut off the Colon Corruptors' food supply by eliminating sugar, fungi, molds, and the products of undesirable fermentation. Now you have those Colon Corruptors on the ropes—they are starving to death while you dine on gut-loving foods. In this chapter, you'll learn how to completely Flush them out with many special foods, herbs, and spices that are tried-and-true nutritional foes of the Colon Corruptors.

As in Week One, you'll keep your gut well Fortified as you continue to avoid sweets, molds, and starches; power up with probiotics and prebiotics; fill up with soluble fiber; include omega-3s in your diet; drink to your health;

and use salt daily. In addition to these Fortification measures, the Gut Flush Plan will add the following six tactics, each specifically designed to Flush any lingering pathogens and parasites from your system.

Flush Tactic #1: Bet on Beta-carotene

Lucky for us, some of brightest, most colorful vegetables—carrots, squash, sweet potatoes, and yams—are also packed with a natural chemical that helps the body defend against pathogens: beta-carotene. This beneficial phytochemical, found in vegetable-based foods, is responsible for that striking orange color on our plates. It also acts as a powerful antioxidant, defusing the destructive power of free radicals, oxidative chemicals that result from exposure to pollutants and to the normal metabolic effects of respiration and energy production.

Scientists are not exactly sure how this conversion works, but it appears beta-carotene is a precursor to vitamin A, a nutrient that helps the body fight off infection. A potent cancer fighter, vitamin A can be dangerous when consumed at high doses in supplement form. That's one of the reasons why the Gut Flush Plan features plenty of foods with beta-carotene, to ensure that you can *safely* get your fill of vitamin A.

Perhaps most important to the Gut Flush Plan, beta-carotene protects the long-term health of the intestinal tract. In studies on animals, researchers have found it limits the development of tumors in the large intestine and helps boost the body's immune defenses. In protecting the lining of your colon, beta-carotene and other carotenoids (such as lycopene, which makes tomatoes red) limit the oxidation of fats in the digestive tract.

But beta-carotene's benefits don't stop there. It also supports the health of your lungs, for example. As you get older, your lungs lose much of their power to move air in and out. Beta-carotene slows this degenerative process, limiting tissue damage caused by free radicals to help keep your breathing strong. Studies also show that the more beta-carotene you consume from foods, the better your chances of resisting age-related macular degeneration, a process that is a major cause of blindness in older people.

On the Gut Flush Plan, you will find a wide array of cooked veggies that are rich in beta-carotene, such as cooked carrots, squash, sweet potatoes, yams, and even greens. Starting this week, I would like you to enjoy at least *two* servings of beta-carotene-rich foods every day.

Flush Tactic #2: Go *Coconutty*!

This week, as in Week One, you'll also continue to take *one tablespoon each of flaxseed and fish oil* every day, to support your cellular membranes. Instead of Week One's olive oil, however, I would like you to use *one tablespoon of coconut oil* several times a week.

Coconut oil contains medium-chain triglycerides (MCTs), which are easier to metabolize than other saturated fatty acids. Plus, these MCTs contain a type of fat called lauric acid, which is both antiviral and antimicrobial—features that fit beautifully with our focus on Flushing this week.

When you eat coconut and coconut oil, you are consuming a major nutritional player in human history. Since the coconut shell forms a wonderful natural, portable container of water and nourishment, it's been carried across the oceans for thousands of years. It has allowed people to go on voyages of exploration, set up long trade routes, and settle in the lands of South America, India, Africa, and the Pacific Rim. Simply loading coconuts on their boats provided the type of dinner boxes (OK, dinner spheres) that could go anywhere. Globally, today more than a billion acres are planted with coconuts.

We humans may love the taste of coconut, but, happily, food-borne pathogens don't. Researchers have found that the lauric acid in coconut oil can wipe out a variety of problematic bacteria, including staph and strep, without ever encountering any resistance.

In the digestive tract, lauric acid is converted into what is called monolaurin, a substance that can kill viruses, pathogenic bacteria (such as Listeria monocytogenes, a common food poisoning agent), and protozoan parasites (such as Giardia lambia, which causes serious diarrhea). Coconut oil has also been shown to kill Candida albicans, chlamydia, and H. pylori. As if these anti–Colon Corruptor actions weren't enough, lab experiments have shown that coconut oil can increase enzyme activity that gives you more personal energy. By activating these enzymes that burn fat, coconut oil may even help you lose weight!

Although coconut is full of saturated fat, it doesn't really harm your heart health. That's because much of its saturated fat consists of that same lauric acid which, research shows, is one of the fats that boost your good HDL cholesterol, the type that helps keep arteries clear of blockages.

Coconut oil is made not just from the milk inside the coconut but results from pressing oils from the meat of the fruit. When buying coconut oil, read the label to make sure it is extra-virgin and not hydrogenated, since hydrogenation adds toxic trans fats (see Chapter 10 for the brand names of the coconut oil that I like best).

Flush Tactic #3: Keep Out the Unfriendly Carbs

Remember that sugars and even hypoallergenic gluten-free grains and starches can provide a food source for yeast and parasites, so moderation is a keynote during Week Two. Having said this, I don't want you to be deprived, as is the case with so many Candida- and parasite-control diets. This is also one of the reasons you will see Follow Your Heart grapeseed-oil Vegenaise on the list. Vegenaise does contain a source of sugar (brown rice syrup); however, it is present in such minute amounts that I am giving it a "pass."

Enjoy up to *two* servings daily of gluten-free grains and starches, such as quinoa, buckwheat, amaranth, brown rice, and millet. The exception would be for those of you who have a very delicate digestive system and would prefer to avoid all grains at this time—which in some individuals can provide a "feeding" source for yeast and other nasty bacteria. Please note you will continue to avoid all fruit and fruit juices as well as all other sweeteners until Week Three.

Flush Tactic #4: Spice Up Your Life

In addition to making food taste downright delicious, many herbs and spices are also powerful weapons against Colon Corruptors. In particular, the Gut Flush Plan makes ample use of cinnamon, garlic, oregano, and cayenne, as these spices are effective at Flushing bugs that give you food poisoning, diarrhea, and even ulcers. As an added bonus, these spices and herbs also have a wide variety of other health benefits.

THE SPECIFIC CARBOHYDRATE DIET

If you suffer from serious digestive problems, such as Crohn's disease, ulcerative colitis, diverticulitis, inflammatory bowel disease, or chronic diarrhea, you may benefit from a slight tweak to the Gut Flush Plan. According to Elaine Gottschall, who developed the Specific Carbohydrate Diet, you can eliminate some of these more serious digestive problems by eating only carbohydrates that are monosaccharides. These types of carbs contain a molecular structure that permits them to be more easily absorbed through the walls of the intestine. Dr. Gottschall argues that with extremely sensitive people who have the above-mentioned disorders, complex carbohydrates—disaccharides with double molecules and polysaccharides made of chained molecules—are not recommended because they remain in the digestive tract too long and feed both yeast and bacteria, which, in turn, form acids and toxins that injure the intestinal lining.

Gottschall's approach is based on these principles:

1. Food contains three classes of sugars: monosaccharides (simple sugars as found in honey, fruits, and some veggies); disaccharides (double sugars found in milk, table sugar, and corn syrup); and polysaccharides (starches found in rice, corn, potatoes, sweet potatoes, yams, and other grains).
2. When disaccharide and polysaccharide sugars enter the GI tract, they must be broken down into monosaccharides before being absorbed.
3. Bacteria in the intestines ferment and feed on the larger sugar molecules (disaccharides and polysaccarides) that linger in the gut.
4. The fermentation of carbohydrates in the intestinal tract leads to the overgrowth of harmful bacteria that damages health and digestion and leads to food intolerances.

When the body lacks the enzyme to break down lactose, a disaccharide milk sugar, this imbalance of bacteria can lead to lactose intolerance. Because undigested lactose stays in the intestines, it serves as a food source for fermenting bacteria. The result: severe stomach pain, diarrhea, and flatulence.

Gottschall's approach can be very helpful to individuals who have had long-

(continued)

standing digestive diseases. If you have any of the conditions mentioned above, you can adapt the Gut Flush Plan accordingly by making some minor adjustments to the three-week menu plan. Just replace some of the more complex carbs (the nongluten grains and starchy vegetables, such as brown rice, amaranth, quinoa, buckwheat, millet, sweet potatoes, and yams) with nonstarchy vegetables (such as summer squash, zucchini, string beans, broccoli, cauliflower, and the like). But please note that this approach does require that you include fruits and honey, two elements that are purposefully omitted from the Gut Flush Plan (fruit for two weeks at least) because they can feed parasites and yeast.

Cinnamon

Consider that hiding behind that subtle sweet and spicy taste, cinnamon is a killer—a killer of pathogens, that is. For instance, cinnamon is lethal against E. coli O157:H7, one of the most problematic bacteria that infect food, as well as Salmonella and campylobacter. When scientists took room temperature apple juice that had about a million E. coli O157:H7 bacteria in it and dropped a teaspoon of cinnamon into this yucky concoction, the cinnamon zapped 99.5 percent of the bacteria in three days. Oh, and by the way, that million E. coli O157:H7 is about *one hundred times* the amount you'd find in food normally contaminated with this bacteria. That's why researchers who have looked into cinnamon's antipathogenic effects recommended that the spice be added to unpasteurized fruit juice.

Cinnamon can also be used to wipe out the pathogenic bacteria in your mouth that can give you bad breath. When researchers investigated the effects of chewing Big Red gum, which contains a cinnamon extract, they found that the cinnamon's cinnamic aldehyde was an effective antimicrobial that killed about half the bad bugs in saliva.

As an added bonus, cinnamon can also help your body handle blood sugar. The cells of people who have type 2 diabetes or who are insulin resistant generally have trouble taking in sugar circulating in the arteries. But laboratory experiments at the U.S. Agricultural Research Service show that cinnamon can get cells to once again recognize the signals from insulin that they should take sugar out of the blood.

Garlic

We may hate the smell of garlic on our breath, but bacteria hate garlic even more. Scientists in Nigeria have found that garlic can destroy the kind of bacteria that would otherwise give you diarrhea. And though it may seem somewhat counterintuitive, garlic has also been found to effectively flush out the bad bacteria in your mouth when used in a mouthwash. Researchers who work in the Food Science unit of the Department of Animals Sciences and Industry at Kansas State University have also found that garlic is effective at zapping antibiotic-resistant Superbugs. And, of course, garlic is a well-respected antiparastic, antifungal, and antiyeast herb.

Oregano

When it comes to rubbing out Superbugs, oregano may be the all-time champion. When researchers at Georgetown University compared oregano's effects with those of antibiotics, they found that oregano more than held its own against Staphylococcus, the source of many drug-resistant infections. Another big advantage oregano boasts is that dangerous pathogens can't develop resistance against its devastating powers. Oregano is a natural antiviral, an anti-inflammatory, and is said to contain the highest amount of antioxidants in the herb kingdom. As we discussed in Chapter 3, oregano is also a well-respected fungus remover.

Cayenne

Chefs in tropical climates have been using cayenne to spice things up for thousands of years. When archaeologists excavated ancient kitchens in the caves of pre-Columbian inhabitants, they found evidence of ten different types of chili peppers being used to prepare food at least fifteen hundred years ago. In Peru, other scientists found chili peppers that were six thousand years old!

The warm temperatures in certain countries encourage the growth of pathogens on food, which is why ancient people relied upon a great deal of cayenne, and why even today it's an amazing killer of bad bugs that would otherwise make us sick. When researchers in Spain treated hamburger with cayenne and then left it out at room temperature for four days, they found the cayenne had killed off bacteria and kept the meat from spoiling as fast as it would have if left on its own.

The active ingredient in hot peppers is capsaicin, which makes your mouth tingle and burn when it touches the sensitive neurons inside your cheeks and on your tongue. In Chapter 5 we talked about how capsaicin has been shown to kill H. pylori, the bacteria that cause stomach ulcers. As an added benefit, it also slows down the inflammation caused by H. pylori. And researchers at Virginia Tech have found that adding capsaicin to the diet of baby chicks makes them more resistant to Salmonella, a common contaminant of chickens. Cayenne helps us resist food poisoning because the capsaicin acts in the intestine to enlist support from the immune cells that can fight off bugs like Salmonella.

If that wasn't enough, lab tests show capsaicin also inhibits the growth of ovarian cancer cells, slowly withers prostate cancer cells, and just downright slaughters pancreatic cancer cells. Creams made with capsaicin relieve pain of osteoarthritis, probably by stimulating nerves to release abundant chemical signals that signify pain so that they run out of signaling material. End result: no more pain. Talk about a hot spice!

On the Gut Flush Plan, you'll enjoy all of these flavorful, therapeutic herbs and spices. During Week Two, you will find oregano and cinnamon on the menu several times a week, and both garlic and cayenne will be used on a daily basis. If you are not going to follow the menu plan and want to try your hand at culinary creativity, consider spicing up your health with oregano in sauces and salad dressings; cinnamon in lamb and chicken dishes; garlic in salsas and casseroles; and cayenne in vegetables and meat dishes.

Flush Tactic #5: Add More Colon Corruptor Killer Foods to Your Diet

Parasites, in particular, do not like certain compounds within pumpkin seeds, kelp, sauerkraut, ground almonds, or radishes, which is why you will see these foods incorporated frequently into the 21-Day Gut Flush Plan. While these foods all have particular properties that make them foes for Colon Corruptors, they each pack additional nutritional punch.

Pumpkin seeds

Traditionally, Native Americans used pumpkin seeds to fight off parasites in the digestive tract and to treat kidney problems. Scientific research has suggested that pumpkin seeds can indeed be useful for intestinal parasites. In Germany, pumpkin seeds are actually used to eliminate tapeworms.

The natural chemicals in pumpkin seeds act as powerful antioxidants in the digestive tract and the blood, fighting off oxidative damage that could harm the digestive tract lining while at the same time helping to protect the liver. And when the oil from pumpkin seeds is given in combination with other herbs to treat type 2 diabetes, it helps lower blood pressure, makes cells more sensitive to insulin, and improves how sugar is metabolized. The oils in pumpkin seeds can even help lower the risk of prostate problems.

Kelp

Kelp enjoys a worldwide reputation for its ability to encourage the digestive tract to expel parasitic worms, and it can also ease irritation of the digestive tract. Kelp is an immune system booster that helps the body fight off infections and parasites. With so many toxins and heavy metals prevalent in our food and environment, it's reassuring to know that kelp can help limit the absorption of these toxins. Kelp even helps fight cancer by lowering levels of estradiol, a hormone linked to breast, endometrial, and ovarian cancers.

Sauerkraut

We talked about the probiotic benefits of sauerkraut in Chapter 7, but sauerkraut has also impressed researchers with its ability to help fight cancer. When cabbage is fermented and yields this tangy food, natural substances called isothiocyanates are formed, and lab tests show that these help prevent tumors. The fact that Polish women, for instance, have a lower rate of breast cancer than their American counterparts is credited to their taste for sauerkraut. Along with isothiocyanates, sauerkraut contains generous amounts of lactic acid, which improves digestion and helps prevent diarrhea.

Almonds

Researchers have found that almonds, especially the skins, have parasite-control benefits. Their vitamin E content along with their flavonoids cooperate synergistically to produce a potent antioxidant effect that may benefit the digestive tract. As a result, almonds may also significantly lower your risk of colon cancer. Almonds are also great for keeping arteries unblocked and they provide more vitamin E than any other nut. They raise good HDL cholesterol and drop bad LDL, and a study in the *Archives of Internal Medicine* found that eating an ounce of almonds a week can reduce your risk of sudden cardiac death by almost 50 percent.

Radishes

Research from Belgium shows radishes contain antifungal compounds that can stop Candida cells from growing. Radishes also contain natural pigments called anthocyanins that can help fight colon cancer. Traditionally, radish is used to overcome intestinal gas and stomachaches while helping to expel digestive worms. Radish also stimulates bile from the liver, aiding digestion, killing bacteria and pathogens, and toning the digestive tract so that food and wastes move through more efficiently.

With the exception of almonds, most of these foods do not find their way into the average American's diet—which is exactly why I've singled out many of them for inclusion in the 21-Day Gut Flush Plan. If you want to simply tweak your current eating plan, then by all means have at least one-quarter to one-half cup ground or whole pumpkin seeds, a dash of kelp granules on your veggies, one-half cup sauerkraut, a handful of almonds, and at least a radish a day to keep parasites away.

Flush Tactic #6: Add Flushing Beverages to Your Day

If staying adequately hydrated was important to Fortifying your body against new attacks, it is absolutely *critical* to helping Flush out any existing pathogens. In addition to continuing to drink *half your body weight in ounces* of water during Week Two, I would like you to add at least *two* cups of a flushing beverage. (This drink will take the place of Week One's Fortifying beverages). Choose from Pau d'Arco (also known as Taheebo) and/or mugwort tea.

Pau d'Arco

Made from the bark of the of Amazonian rain forest *Tabebuia avellanedae* tree, Pau d'Arco tea has been used for medicinal purposes for hundreds, if not thousands, of years to treat ailments from arthritis and cancer to fever and boils. Since the early 1960s, medical experiments have indicated that Pau d'Arco can offset pain, act as a diuretic, limit psoriasis, and help lower the risk of cancer, all while killing viruses, bacteria, and fungus.

It is not clear exactly which of the natural chemicals in the plant is most effective at killing pathogens. As a group, the chemicals in Pau d'Arco's bark that seem to be medicinally effective are called naphthoquinones. Recent studies found that napthoquinones can limit the growth of H. pylori, and while these chemicals were not as effective as certain antibiotics, they did have fewer side effects. Plus, other investigators have found evidence that Pau d'Arco can be effective against Superbugs, particularly methicillin-resistant Staphylococcus aureus (MRSA), the staph infection that is continuing to spread around the world. But rather than seek to isolate the most effective compounds, many researchers agree that the unrefined tea made from Pau d'Arco is more effective in killing bacteria and parasites than any of the single chemical extracts.

Practitioners now routinely recommend the tea for Candida albicans, herpes, parasites like chistosomiasis, brucellosis (a bacterial infection), arthritis, and inflammations of the cervix and vagina. In helping with these conditions, Pau d'Arco enhances immunity, helps the body eliminate toxins, and encourages the production of extra red blood cells that boost oxygen circulation and accelerate healing. A group of Korean researchers who studied the Pau d'Arco believe compounds from the tea even have the potential to be "chemopreventive agents" that can stop the growth of liver and lung cancer cells. Not bad for a simple cup of warm tea.

Mugwort

Mugwort hardly sounds like a serious name for a beneficial herb, but this tea has been used for generations to kill intestinal parasites and worms. Long known to contain chemicals that repel pesky moths, mugwort's name is actually believed to be a derivative of the Old English word *moughte,* meaning "moth."

For many years, herbalists have used mugwort to fight sexually transmitted disease, and recent tests show that compounds in this herb can halt growth of herpesvirus and stop it from spreading from cell to cell. In the past, mugwort was also given to soothe "hysteria," and today the herb is still known for its gentle, sedative powers. For example, mugwort is frequently used as a tonic that can relieve digestive stress. It can also ease aching muscles, or PMS or menstrual complaints, and is a popular ingredient in hot, relaxing baths. Traditionally, in Asia and Europe, mugwort has been given to people complaining of gout and rheumatoid arthritis. If you have any of these conditions, not only will a nice warm cup of mugwort help relieve your symptoms, it will also help Flush out your GI tract.

> *Every tissue in the body is fed by the bloodstream, which is supplied by the bowel. When the bowel is dirty, the blood is dirty, and so are the organs and tissues. It is the bowel that must be cared for first. Sickness and disease respond more effectively and faster to treatment when bowel irrigation is done first.*

—BERNARD JENSEN, alternative health expert who revolutionized our ideas about bowel health and author of *Dr. Jensen's Guide to Better Bowel Care.*

EXTRA FLUSHING FOR YOUR COLON: COLONIC IRRIGATIONS

A series of colonics, also known as high colonics or high enemas, are wonderful adjuncts to the Gut Flush Plan. A colonic involves irrigating the entire length of the large intestine or colon with a lukewarm water solution. The solution is able to gently and effectively dislodge and remove toxins from hard-to-reach pockets where fecal matter tends to accumulate. The procedure takes about forty-five minutes and is usually conducted in a health professional's office by a certified colon hydrotherapist.

Do make sure that your colon hydrotherapist uses water that has been filtered to remove chemicals, heavy metals, and parasites. Also be mindful that additional antiseptic measures, such as disposable speculums, should be used. Finally, an implant of the beneficial bacteria (or probiotics) is the last requirement so that you can reestablish healthy bowel flora once again.

If your colon hydrotherapist is not equipped for implants, then do them yourself after each colonic. Simply use one teaspoon of the powdered probiotic Flora-Key (see Resources) in eight ounces of water and pour into an empty Fleet's enema bottle. Bend over and insert the solution. Try to hold for at least ten to fifteen minutes without eliminating in the bathroom. That's all there is to it.

Many seasoned hydrotherapists believe that a colonic can accurately eliminate volumes of impacted material and excess mucus as well as pathogenic bacteria, parasites, and worms. Many therapists can accurately identify what is passing through the discharge tubing and thereby help you find the correct program and products for your condition.

Experts also believe that colonics, through the gentle internal massage of the water pressure, help to reestablish the original shape of the colon. Bulges and pockets, where wastes and other critters have been "hiding" and fermenting or putrifying, are re-formed back into their healthy shape. In addition, colonics firm up the colon's muscles, stimulating their peristaltic action that squeezes and excretes waste material. In that way, they boost regular bowel movements and put a stop to both constipation and diarrhea.

Sometimes a colon hydrotherapist will suggest a series of colonics based upon your performance and the contents of the material coming out of your body. This series is best done during the spring and fall, which are considered the most opportune times to detox and cleanse. But should you be in need of a colonic between these times, not to worry. I, for one, am a big believer having been a fan of colonics for more than three decades. They literally saved my life.

You've completed the first two transitional weeks of the Gut Flush Plan. By now you're probably feeling more energetic, with greater mental clarity as your GI tract settles down and your system is cleansed of backed-up toxins and waste. No wonder you were feeling sluggish. Perhaps that toxic state of impaired digestion, bloating, irritability, mental fog, and food reactions, such

EXTRA FLUSHING FOR YOUR COLON, PART 2: ENEMAS

If you are the do-it-yourself type, enemas will probably be right up your alley (so to speak). Whereas colonics can cleanse the entire length of the large intestine, all five and a half feet, enemas reach only the lower twelve and a half inches of the colon—but that may be enough for you.

When preparing an enema, use only properly filtered water or distilled water. Sterilize your water to eliminate parasites and pathogens by boiling at a rolling boil for at least ten minutes. Sterilize the tubing and enema bag by soaking them for ten minutes in a diluted Clorox bath (a half teaspoon of Clorox in a gallon of water). Rinse with sterilized water. Now you are ready to insert the tube for the enema.

Adding garlic juice to an enema increases its parasite-proofing power. Garlic supports the normal acidity of the colon. (To kill pinworms in kids, mash two garlic cloves, boil in six ounces of milk and let it cool. Use this for three nights in a row for children with worms.)

Vinegar enemas are also an effective cleansing agent. Simply add two tablespoons of apple cider vinegar to one quart of water.

Blackstrap molasses enemas can pull encrusted fecal matter and parasites off the colon lining and seem to relax the colon. Add one tablespoon of molasses to a quart of water.

---

as headaches and skin problems, is already on its way out and you are experiencing firsthand that health begins in a Fortified and Flushed colon. Now it's time to heal your digestive system and repair any damage that may have been inflicted upon you by the Colon Corruptors. In the next chapter, you'll learn how to Feed your GI tract the foods and supplements it needs to soothe the lining of the stomach and the intestines. You'll regenerate and rejuvenate not only your digestive system but your immunity as well.

Step 3: Feed

YOU ARE NOW READY FOR WEEK THREE OF THE 21-DAY GUT FLUSH Plan. You have successfully Fortified and Flushed and are now ready to Feed your body with the healthiest foods that will draw and build on the success of the previous two weeks. You'll also expand your culinary horizons and enjoy a wider variety of foods. During this week you'll finish building a nutritional foundation that will last a lifetime.

The menu plan in Week Three is really the model for how I would like you to use the Gut Flush Plan for life. This week we'll be adding certain key foods back into your diet. For example, as long as you've taken measures to eradicate the Colon Corruptors and you remain vigilant for signs of future infestations or sensitivities, fruits and starches do have a place in your world— just a very conscious and deliberate place, which we'll define below.

By following the model of this week, you'll automatically include all your previous Fortifying tactics, to support your GI Good Guys, and Flushing tactics, to continually rid your body of Colon Corruptors. In addition, you'll be Feeding the beleaguered lining of your GI tract all the foods it will need to help it heal and regenerate. You'll give your immune system some much-needed nourishment and help it get back in fighting form. Ultimately, when you follow the blueprint for this week's eating plan, you'll help ensure radiant health for your digestive system and your entire body, for life.

Let's look closely at the five specific tactics that help Feed the GI tract the nutrients it needs to sustain and continually improve your long-term health.

Feed Tactic #1: Promote Protein

Very important to Feeding your gut, proteins make up the building blocks of the body, the raw material the body uses to build tissues and organs. Researchers have even found that the body uses specialized proteins to protect the digestive tract. For example, the body converts some of the protein you eat into versatile compounds called lectins. A particular class of lectins is produced by the lining of the intestines to kill bacteria that might otherwise invade the body. They do this by latching on to the sugars in the membranes of bacteria and subsequently ripping apart the pathogens. One researcher refers to these proteins as "killers with a sweet tooth."

Proteins can also stop pathogens and parasites from entering the bloodstream, minimizing the inflammation that creates spaces in the intestinal wall. In a study of one hundred women in Australia who were trying to lose weight, scientists found that eating a high-protein diet decreased inflammation in their bodies (including intestinal inflammation) and improved their blood cholesterol.

While proteins literally make up the wall of the intestine—as they are the raw matter from which the body rebuilds the gastrointestinal tract—they can also limit muscle loss. This trick is equally essential to preserving good digestion.

It goes like this: your body performs most of its muscle-building chores soon after you eat. Every time you consume protein in a meal, you produce double the muscle that you do between meals. However, as you age, this process gradually slows, and it becomes less effective at replacing lost lean tissue as the decades pass. By the time you enter middle age, in your early forties, you can start losing up to 2 percent of your muscle every year.

Research at the Human Nutrition Research Center of Auvergne, INRA, Clermont-Ferrand, France, shows that getting plenty of protein, including the amino acid leucine, can help rebalance this process. If you can prevent the loss of muscle, you can protect that precious smooth muscle in the intestinal wall that propels food down the GI tract. (Whey is one of the richest sources of leucine, which is one of the reasons whey is a part of the Gut Flush Plan.)

Other research confirms the muscle-preserving benefits of protein. When scientists at the University of Illinois, Urbana-Champaign, fed a dozen overweight women high-protein diets for ten weeks, they found that not only did the women lose an average of fifteen pounds (mostly fat), but they also retained more muscle than did dieting women who ate high-carbohydrate diets. Interestingly, other data show that the more thoroughly you chew your food, the better your body can use the protein in your meals for building muscle and other organs.

To ensure that your body gets the protein it needs to rebuild your intestinal tract on the Gut Flush Plan, you'll eat *at least eight ounces of protein per day*, chosen from lean beef, poultry, and fish. To this, you can add *one to two omega-rich eggs* for extra protein snacks. Enjoy *up to two whey-based protein drinks* in addition to the basic protein requirement. Most individuals with lactose or casein allergies can tolerate the Fat Flush whey protein (see Resources), as it is both lactose- and casein-free.

Feed Tactic #2: Vitalize with Veggies

Despite its significant benefits, protein is not the be-all and end-all for gut health—far from it. Consider the case of Amanda.

When Amanda came to meet with me, she was suffering from an uncomfortable, embarrassing case of gas, bloating, and constipation. She was also concerned about her lack of energy and the fact that her skin had begun to suffer with acne and rashes. When I asked her what kind of food she tended to eat, she said she followed a pretty strict high-protein diet to keep her weight down.

While her weight was normal, the total lack of fruits and vegetables in her diet, along with her list of symptoms, showed me that her colon was quickly becoming clogged and toxic. The fact that there were many vitamins, minerals, and antioxidants absent from her diet, as well as little fiber, was keeping her body from properly disposing of toxins.

After I got her started on the Gut Flush Plan, her results were astonishing.

Her colon began functioning normally; her constipation cleared; her energy level zoomed. Happily, she was able to control her weight without even trying, and she was once again able to *crunch* into foods—a satisfying feeling that you just can't get from most protein foods.

Not only is a diet heavy in vegetables good for your complexion and your waistline, but it also provides natural protection against food-borne parasites and other infectious agents. That's because vegetables naturally have protective compounds that they create to ward off pathogens and infections that might kill them, even when they're still growing in the ground.

When researchers at Cornell looked into why vegetarian foods stay fresh longer than meat dishes, even without adding spices or other preservatives, they found that the tissue and muscle that make up meat are defended against infection by an animal's immune system—and that protection abruptly stops functioning when the animal is slaughtered. That's the main reason why traditional meat recipes of cultures in tropical climates tend to contain plenty of antimicrobial spices. When the Cornell scientists measured temperature and rainfall, and the distribution of more than forty spice plants and their antipathogenic properties, they found that the primary function of spicing food in a hot climate was not necessarily for taste but to stop the growth of bacteria, fungi, and parasites.

In contrast, vegetables are safer precisely because they *don't* have the kind of active immune systems that animals have. As a result, vegetables have to rely on phytochemicals, natural substances that kill off bugs, as well as thicker cell walls to keep pathogens at bay. Fortunately for those of us who Feed our GI tract with vegetables, those defensive mechanisms remain in force when we eat produce items. That's why, after you swallow vegetables, these antipathogen natural weapons continue to perform their antipathogen tasks in your digestive system, making it less hospitable to infection. As an added bonus, vegetarian foods have a lower acidity level that's less welcoming to infectious organisms.

When food-borne infections spread, usually some kind of meat dish is to blame as the original source of food poisoning. And while this isn't always the case—as evidenced by recalls of spinach and other produce contaminated with E. coli—there are still many more recalls of foods such as hamburger meat than there are vegetarian foods. So bring on the veggies.

On the Gut Flush Plan, you'll enjoy *at least five vibrant nonstarchy veggies per day*, such as asparagus, zucchini, tomatoes, parsley, yellow squash, broccoli, cauliflower, red, green, and yellow bell peppers, and many other delicious varieties.

Feed Tactic #3: Sweeten Up with Fruits

By eliminating fruits during weeks One and Two, you gave your body a better chance to Fortify against and Flush out yeast and other undesirables in the digestive tract. But once you have regained some of your intestinal fortitude, you can reintroduce a limited amount of fruit, which will allow you to take in more of the valuable natural chemicals that the body uses in its immune defenses.

Just like vegetables, fruits are also packed with phytochemicals that may help the body stop the growth of pathogens, parasites, and undesirable bacteria. While their sugar content, if you consume too many fruits, may sometimes encourage the growth of yeast, the fiber and phytochemicals in fruit offer dependable benefits to the body's disease-fighting processes. They may also lower your risk of cancer and heart disease. And more good news: many fruits and other vegetarian foods contain oleanolic acid and derivatives of this chemical that act as natural protectors against pathogens.

Other beneficial phytochemicals form in ripening fruits in a way that's similar to the process that turns leaves their fall colors. Just as leaves are green in the summer because of the dominant coloring of chlorophyll, unripe fruits are greenish because of their chlorophyll content. When fruits ripen, however, the chlorophyll breaks down, the same way it breaks down in the leaves. Scientists at the University of Innsbruck in Austria have discovered that in the peels of fruits, chlorophyll is converted into powerful antioxidants called nonfluorescing chlorophyll catabolytes. The researchers think these chemicals play a large role in protecting the health of the GI tract and the entire body.

When fruits are cooked, some of their natural enzymes are broken down, but other nutrients, like carotenoids, may become more available for absorption. For example, when you cook tomatoes, you enhance the amount of lycopene you take in. Lycopene has been linked to a lower risk of various cancers.

While all sugars and fruits are omitted during weeks One and Two of the Gut Flush Plan, during Week Three you can now rotate back *up to two fruits per day*, which are perfect choices for smoothies or snacks. Choose from the low-sugar but satisfying apple (1), pear (1), berries (1 cup), plum (2), peach (1), nectarine (1), cherries (10), grapefruit (½), orange (1), avocado (½). (If diarrhea is still a challenge, please cook your fruits!) Also note that for variety you can substitute half of a fruit exchange for one fruit juice–sweetened slice of bread or waffle. The shopping list has many gluten-free and fruit juice–sweetened choices.

Feed Tactic #4: Satisfy with Starches

Thus far, we've been very conservative with starches on the Gut Flush Plan. This week we'll further broaden our food palette. Besides the colorful squashes, sweet potato, and yams you've enjoyed previously, you can now also *eat beans several times a week.*

Beans and humans have a long history together. They were among the first plants that people grew for food. Archaeologists have found beans among the pyramids of Egypt and in the Western Hemisphere. One huge advantage of beans is their high-protein content. One cup of beans contains about a quarter of your daily protein needs. That's probably why armies throughout history have lived on beans—they're a cheap, durable, portable source of plentiful nutrition. Beans are also rich in phytochemicals that reduce your risk of heart disease. These phytochemicals, classified as phytoestrogens (plant estrogens), improve blood cholesterol, help arteries relax, and keep blood pressure down.

One of the primary benefits of beans and other legumes, such as lentils and peas, for Feeding and maintaining the health of the digestive tract is the fact that they contain what is called resistant starch. Resistant starch "resists digestion" as it travels through much of the GI tract, moving through the stomach and small intestine mostly intact until it reaches the colon. Once it reaches the lower part of the digestive tract, resistant starch provides nutrition for probiotic bacteria, which convert much of it to butyrate—a short-chain fatty acid that lowers the risk of cancer while it provides the nutrition that the intestines use to rebuild and repair themselves.

Butyrate is so powerful at stimulating intestinal repair that medical researchers have given this substance intravenously to hospital patients who have had sections of the small intestine surgically removed. In these tests, butyrate caused the intestine to grow back and made the remaining sections more functional. Scientists have also discovered that butyrate increases the size and effectiveness of the villi in the intestines, the fingerlike projections in the intestinal tract that are responsible for picking out nutrients and absorbing them into the bloodstream. Some people with Crohn's disease who were totally reliant on intravenous feeding because their intestines were so compromised found that butyrate helped them regain the ability to eat food by mouth again.

Beans also contain large amounts of regular dietary fiber as well as resistant starch. Black beans, in particular, are high in both dietary fiber and resistant starch. But if your GI tract is having a serious problem with an imbalance of infectious agents like Candida, beans' starch may feed the undesirable pathogens. That's why I don't recommend beans right at the beginning of the Gut Flush Plan. They need to be reintroduced gradually as you make progress in Feeding and fixing your gut.

Garbanzos, adzuki, black beans, and lentils are especially high in minerals. Just remember that the harder beans must be presoaked for twenty-four hours to remove starchy residues that can create digestive discomfort.

Feed Tactic #5: Add a Feeding Beverage

Beyond consuming half of your body weight in ounces of water during the day, I would like you to make a tea out of the healing/soothing slippery elm powder. Simply empty four capsules into a mug and add one cup of boiling water, stirring constantly until the powder dissolves. Aim for *at least two cups of slippery elm tea per day.*

Traditionally, slippery elm has been one of the herbs most frequently used to soothe inflammatory bowel disease. In particular, it has been employed in both traditional Chinese medicine and Ayurvedic medicine for alleviating gastrointestinal complaints like diarrhea. Long a standard herbal remedy used by Native Americans, slippery elm was used for a wide range of complaints, including boils, wounds, ulcer, skin inflammation, chapped lips, arthritic pain, burns, cough, and even as a cure for chapped lips. In an early foreshadowing of its role in Gut Flush, slippery elm was the helpful remedy Native Americans shared with early American colonists to relieve some of their most troubling maladies: kidney problems, hemorrhoids, constipation, and diarrhea.

Slippery elm's benefits are believed to derive from the fact that it is a demulcent: when mixed with water, it forms a mucilaginous oily residue that can soothe irritations and may keep toxins and microbes from coming in contact with the mucosal lining of the gastrointestinal tract. Slippery elm can also speed the passage of wastes through the digestive tract, helping to eliminate toxins and pathogens. Plus, because it forms bulk in the colon, it may retain toxins that might otherwise be absorbed through the walls of the large intestine. Because of those characteristics, and the fact that you can eat this herb in relatively large quantities, it is particularly useful in coating and soothing the digestive tract.

While the slippery elm can be taken as a capsule, it may also be made into a porridge similar in consistency to oatmeal. Herbalists sometimes recommend eating it three times a day to ease gastritis and other intestinal complaints. Along with its physically soothing characteristics, recent lab tests confirm that slippery elm contains antioxidants that might help heal intestinal inflammations. Please be sure to enjoy the soothing, healing properties of slippery elm in your own gut.

Feed Tactic #6: Repair Your Gut with L-glutamine and Gamma Oryzanol

Two additional supplements can help speed the repair of your gut and heal any damage in the mucosal lining of the GI tract. Both L-glutamine, an amino acid, and gamma oryzanol, a powerful antioxidant, help rebuild the muscle tissue that can be damaged by Colon Corruptors. In Week Three, you'll add 500–3,000 mg of L-glutamine between meals (I prefer Carlson's powdered L-glutamine) as well as approximately 380 mg deglycyrrhized licorice (DGL) twenty minutes before meals three times daily. Let's look at why.

L-glutamine

Also found in muscle tissue, the brain, the lungs, and the liver, L-glutamine is present in large amounts in the lining of the digestive tract. When muscles or the lining of the intestinal tract are damaged, glutamine plays a vital role in the process that fixes the damage.

Researchers have found that giving glutamine helps maintain the proper permeability of the small intestines. Without glutamine, the villi (the parts of the small intestines that allow nutrients in) become too porous. Molecules enter that body that normally would be too large to breach the intestinal wall. That results in substances being allowed into the bloodstream that can cause allergic reactions and other problematic responses. On the other hand, glutamine helps the lining allow the proper nutrients into the body while barring the entry of allergens.

Along with allergens, when your intestinal tract is damaged or stressed, microbes and the toxins they secrete can also find their way through the intestinal walls and lead to infection. Here, too, glutamine helps keep these nasty substances out by aiding in creating a barrier that protects the body. In addition, the cells of the intestinal walls responsible for choosing which nutrients are permitted into the body are fueled by glutamine.

Researchers have found that besides Feeding the cells in the intestines and helping put up barriers to pathogens, glutamine helps boost the growth of probiotics, which in turn also help defend the intestinal walls against pathogenic invasion. When researchers gave glutamine to people with ulcerative colitis, they found that it reduced intestinal inflammation—and their probiotic bacteria flourished as well. It works best one or two hours before or after meals because acids destroy its activity.

As an added feel-better bonus, L-glutamine also Feeds the immune cells that dwell in the intestinal tract. When researchers in Poland gave glutamine to a dozen hospital patients with damaged intestinal tracts who were malnourished and getting weaker, they found that this versatile amino acid revived many of their lymphocytes (cells that take part in the immune system) and improved their absorption of protein and other nutrients.

DGL

DGL (deglycyrrhized licorice) is a centuries-old, highly effective therapy used to heal gastritis and ulcers. For more than forty years, various medical journals have sung the praises of DGL, which enhances the production of healing mucus, unlike medications used for gastritis. It is also a potent anti-inflammatory with antioxidant properties that stimulates healing with damaged mucous membranes.

DGL is a wonderful promoter of salivary compounds that trigger benefi-

COFFEE ENEMAS

As you know by now, I am not a big fan of coffee—that is, when it's taken in the usual way. But coffee enemas are a different story. In a sense, a coffee enema "feeds" the liver and gallbladder. The result is a purging of toxic bile, which then helps to clear out the lower colon as well as the liver and gallbladder—three organs cleaned out with a simple enema. You might wish to do this procedure at least twice during Week Three.

For this treatment, you will need a coffeemaker, organic ground coffee, four emptied Fleet enemas, and a lubricant like natural cocoa butter.

Take the enema after a bowel movement rather than before one. Many people prefer to do this procedure while lying down on an old towel or blanket on the bathroom floor. Some bring pillows, books, or magazines. Then follow these steps:

1. Place about four to six tablespoons of ground coffee in the coffee filter. Pour one quart of pure water through the filter.
2. Cool the coffee to room temperature.
3. Fill each of the Fleet enemas with the coffee.
4. Insert each one by lubricating the tip with the cocoa butter.
5. Gently massage your abdomen for five minutes while lying on your left side. Do the same thing while lying on your back, and then on your right side.
6. After fifteen minutes (or as long as you can hold it), sit on the toilet and expel the enema. Remember that you should never try to forcibly hold in the enema. In fact, nothing in this entire procedure should involve force or strain.

cial growth and rejuvenation of both intestinal and stomach cells. DGL is very helpful when mixed with saliva, so chewing tablets is ideal.

You are now armed with all the knowledge you'll need to begin the Gut Flush Plan and make the successful transition to a clean, pathogen-free, and revitalized digestive system—as well as a whole new way of life. If you are eager to begin the plan, turn to the next chapter for all the help you need to prepare your mind, body, and—perhaps most important—your kitchen to get flushed.

PART

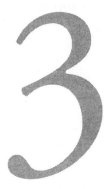

The 21-Day
Gut Flush Plan

10

Getting Ready for Gut Flush

THE BEAUTY OF THE GUT FLUSH PLAN IS THAT FINALLY YOU WILL HAVE the chance to get off your Gut Grief merry-go-round once and for all. You'll be venturing out into a whole new world of eating, one that focuses on foods that are brimming with flavor and bursting with health benefits. I promise you won't even miss all that sugar, yeast, wheat, and corn because you will be so thrilled with a smoothly functioning digestive tract and the absence of gas, bloating, various assorted aches and pains, and even food cravings. Yes, you can expect to lose a pound or two or even more—almost effortlessly. Weight loss is a frequently reported side effect of eating the Gut Flush way.

Now, before you begin the 21-day plan to Fortify, Flush, and Feed your gut, I'd like you to prepare just a few things, in order for you to get the most out of the program. First, designate a day to start your program, so you can gear yourself up mentally and get all your supplies in order. Give yourself at least three to four days to prepare and stock your house (maybe more, if you need to special-order any products). I'd like you to have everything necessary in your home and ready, so that from the very first day, you'll get the maximum benefit out of the plan.

Preparing for the plan entails three stages: stocking your kitchen; establishing a pure water source; and creating your Gut Flush Food Journal. Because readying your kitchen with the best foods is the easiest way to ensure your success on the plan, let's start there first.

Stocking the Gut Flush Kitchen

To get ready for this program, make certain that your fridge, freezer, and pantry are well supplied with the right staples so you can be completely supported in your Gut Flushing efforts. This section will contain a complete shopping list of *nonperishable* foods for all three weeks of the plan. This allows you to easily purchase all your pantry staples in one trip. Separate shopping lists for the *perishables* can be found following each week's meal plan.

I think you will continually be amazed to learn that Gut Flush eating is not as restrictive as you may have thought. Actually, there are plenty of delicious and appealing foods that meet all of the criteria, as you will soon find out. Many of the foods itemized below can be found in "enlightened" grocery stores these days, as well as in whole foods–based supermarkets. Brand names are included for your convenience, and many of them are ones that I use in my own home. Of course, there are numerous others that may qualify as well— all you have to do is start reading labels.

I have also included some items (like the frozen tricolor peppers, for example) that are not on the 21-Day Gut Flush Plan. I want you to have plenty of variety to choose from in case you aren't a fan of the featured veggie of the meal.

You will be happy to note that although you may be going gluten-free for a while, you don't have to give up bread entirely. One standout product: Kinnikinnik Candadi yeast-free multigrain rice bread makes the best toast and sandwiches. And I guarantee you won't miss regular pasta after you have sampled Nutrition Kitchen's whole soybean pasta; not only is it tasty, but it is also loaded with lots more protein (23 grams in two ounces of one-quarter package) than the white or whole wheat stuff.

Do opt for organic whenever possible. Even when I'm eating organic foods, I still use the Gut Flush Food Bath (see page 37) for all my meats, poultry, fish, eggs, and produce to protect against pathogenic bacteria.

Here's what you will need to fill the Gut Flush Kitchen fridge, freezer, and pantry in order to get you on your way to a healthier and more vital you.

The Gut Flush Equipment

Meat thermometer (I prefer a dial-read rather than digital), Misto oil mister, Reynold's parchment paper, vegetable steamer (a nice addition, but not required).

GUT FLUSH TIP • Look for the meat thermometer, oil mister, and vegetable steamer at stores such as Bed Bath and Beyond, Linens 'n Things, Wal-Mart, or a restaurant-supply store. Reynold's parchment paper can be found in your local supermarket.

The Gut Flush Fridge

OILS: Omega Nutrition flaxseed oil, Carlson's Very Finest Fish Oil (lemon flavor), Lucinni's and Spectrum organic olive oil, Spectrum organic sesame oil, Nutiva organic extra-virgin coconut oil, Follow Your Heart grapeseed-oil Vegenaise (has a negligible amount of brown rice syrup).

GUT FLUSH TIP • Store oils in a cool, dark, and dry environment to prevent rancidity. Flaxseed oil is especially subject to oxidation, is sensitive to light, heat, and air, and has a shorter "shelf life." Always store in the fridge and use in about three weeks. Mayos, of course, must be stored in fridge after opening.

SEEDS, NUTS, AND NUT BUTTERS: Cold milled flaxseed (Omega Nutrition or Health from the Sun's FiProFlax), sesame seeds, pumpkin seeds, walnuts, Brazil nuts, almonds, filberts, pecans, macadamia nuts, pine nuts, almond butter, and tahini (Arrowhead Mills Woodstock Farms almond and sesame [tahini] butters).

GUT FLUSH TIP • Nuts may be stored for longer periods of time in the freezer to prolong their freshness.

PROTEIN FOODS: Tofu (firm and/or soft) and tempeh (Mori-Nu and White Wave), eggs (omega-3-enriched such as Eggland's Best, Born 3, Organic Valley, and Pilgrim's Pride Eggs Plus).

GUT FLUSH TIP • Storing perishable protein foods at a temperature below 40 degrees Fahrenheit is essential to inhibit the growth of bacteria. Refrigerate or freeze these foods immediately after purchase. Do keep in mind that meats such as beef and poultry may be stored in the fridge for just two days—that's why I've included them below in the freezer section. The recommended fridge time for storing seafood of any kind is just twenty-four hours.

PROBIOTICS: Organic plain kefir (Lifeway, Helios), organic plain yogurts (Nancy's, Stonyfield, Cascade, Brown Cow, Seven Stars, Horizon), organic brown, red, or yellow miso (Eden, Westbrae), organic sauerkraut (Eden, Rejuvenative).

GUT FLUSH TIP • The kefir and yogurt should always be refrigerated, but the miso and sauerkraut (unless you have a refrigerated brand) can remain in the pantry until opened.

DAIRY: Butter, cream (Horizon), ghee (Purity Farms clarified butter).

GUT FLUSH TIP • Although I mentioned it before, it doesn't hurt to reiterate that fats such as butter, cream, and ghee are not digested like milk or cheese. Many individuals who are sensitive to the lactose and casein in milk and the casein in cheese do just fine with dairy fats.

VEGETABLES: Jerusalem artichokes, leeks, shallots,* onions,* chives, scallions, garlic,* jicama, asparagus, broccoli, beets, artichokes, Brussels sprouts, cabbage, Eden Organic sauerkraut, cucumbers, celery, cauliflower, radishes (red and daikon), chili peppers, sweet red, orange, yellow, and green peppers, leaf lettuces, arugula, radicchio, escarole, endive, watercress, spinach, greens (kale, collards, mustard, beet, dandelion, Swiss chard), sprouts (mung bean, alfalfa, red clover, broccoli), green beans, tomatoes, turnips, rutabagas, okra, kohlrabi, parsnips, carrots, peas (sugar snap, snow, garden, lima), eggplant, bok choy, tomatillos, rhubarb, jalapenos, water chestnuts, rhubarb, squash (both summer—zucchini, crookneck—and winter—spaghetti, delicata, kobocha, acorn, butternut, pumpkin, buttercup, etc.*), sweet potatoes and yams.

GUT FLUSH TIP • Starred (*) vegetables should be stored in the pantry in a cool, dry place and once cut, wrapped and refrigerated. Always try to eat organic foods, which have fewer pesticide residues. Take part in Consumer Supported Agriculture (CSA), which connects you to local organic farmers in your area, ensuring you the safest produce while also helping protect your community's natural environment. (Find information at www.localharvest.org/csa.)

FRUITS: Apples, avocados, seasonal berries (raspberries, blackberries, blueberries, strawberries, cranberries, etc.), pomegranates, nectarines, plums, peaches, grapefruit, oranges, pears, cherries, limes, and lemons.

GUT FLUSH TIP • After purchase, if ripening of fruit is still necessary, keep at room temperature. Once fruit has reached desired ripeness, refrigerate. Berries would be an exception to this recommendation; refrigerate after purchase.

FRESH HERBS: Basil, cilantro, tarragon, parsley, thyme, rosemary, sage, lemongrass, ginger, savory, bay leaves, marjoram, oregano, fennel, dill, mint.

GUT FLUSH TIP • Fresh herbs are very perishable and proper handling is needed to make them last. Store bunches of herbs with their stems in fresh water. Leaves should be kept in the coldest part of your refrigerator in bags with holes. Herbs may be slightly damp, but too much moisture promotes decay. Salad spinners are a great way to dry herbs. I also recommend placing a paper towel in the bag with the herbs to absorb excess water.

BROTHS: Chicken, beef, and vegetable broths (Pacific, Imagine, Health Valley).

GUT FLUSH TIP • Refrigerate opened boxes or cans of broth for no longer than four days. Have extra broth you don't want to throw away? Simply freeze broth in ice cube trays, which can be popped out as needed for quick stir-fries.

ALMOND AND RICE MILKS: Unsweetened almond and rice milks (Pacific, Imagine).

GUT FLUSH TIP • These milks can be stored in the pantry until they are opened. Leftovers need to be refrigerated.

The Gut Flush Freezer

GLUTEN-FREE BREADS: Breads (Food for Life brown rice bread, rice almond bread, rice pecan bread; Kinnikinnick Candida yeast-free multigrain rice bread).

GUT FLUSH TIP • I like to store all my breads in the freezer, which seems to prolong their "freshness." Toasting these breads really brings out the flavor.

OTHER GLUTEN-FREE GRAINS: Waffles (Van's wheat-free flax waffles, wheat-free original waffles, wheat-free cinnamon apple waffles, wheat-free blueberry waffles), pizza crust (Nature's Hilights organic brown rice pizza crust).

GUT FLUSH TIP • Top your pizza crusts with lots of good sauce and veggies.

FROZEN VEGETABLES: Mixed veggies, asparagus, green beans, edamame (green soy beans), peas, tricolor peppers, spinach, broccoli, cauliflower, carrots, lima beans, snap peas (Cascade or Woodstock Organic).

GUT FLUSH TIP • Make sure opened bags of frozen vegetables are closed tightly to prevent freezer burn. To prevent having excess leftovers, add vegetables to soups, stews, and stir-fries.

FROZEN FRUITS: Unsweetened mixed berries, strawberries, blackberries, blueberries, raspberries, peaches, cherries (Cascade, Woodstock Farms Organic), cranberries (available seasonally).

GUT FLUSH TIP • As with opened bags of veggies, make sure bags of frozen fruit are closed tightly to prevent freezer burn. Use small quantities of fruit in muffins, breads, and smoothies.

PROTEIN FOODS: Ground turkey, turkey sausage, and Italian sausage (Shelton), turkey burgers (Applegate Farms organic 100% turkey burgers), chicken breasts, stew meat, steaks, ground sirloin, wild-caught salmon, tuna steaks, shrimp, scallops, ground lamb and lamb chops, turkey breast.

• Choose organic meats whenever possible for their higher quality and lack of added hormones and chemicals.

The Gut Flush Pantry

DRIED HERBS AND SPICES: Anise, arrowroot, cayenne, celery seed, cinnamon, black mustard seeds, mustard powder, garlic powder, coriander, cumin, fennel seeds, ginger, nutmeg, cloves, turmeric, bay leaves, oregano, basil, thyme, rosemary, dill, parsley, sage, marjoram, tarragon, allspice, saffron, Chinese five-spice powder (Simply Organic, Frontier, Spice Hunter).

GUT FLUSH TIP • Choose nonirradiated organic herbs and spices whenever possible for their higher quality and lack of added chemicals.

GLUTEN-FREE PASTA: Various pasta shapes and brands, including Ancient Harvest quinoa and Heartland's Finest pastas (all shapes), Tinkyada brown rice pasta (all shapes), Lundberg Family Farms organic brown rice pasta (all shapes), Pastariso rice pasta, Nutrition Kitchen organic whole golden or green soybean pasta.

GUT FLUSH TIP • You can find many of these pastas at www.wheatfreepasta .com.

GLUTEN-FREE GRAINS: Quinoa, amaranth, buckwheat (Ancient Harvest or Arrowhead Mills), and various rices (Lundberg Family Farms brown, wild, Wehani and Wild Blends; Lotus Foods Forbidden Rice and Bhutanese Red Rice—beautiful color!—Lowell Farms organic brown jasmine rice; unseasoned brown basmati or wild rices; Shiloh Farms millet).

GUT FLUSH TIP • Organic gluten-free grains (particularly rice) can be purchased in bulk at a natural foods market.

GLUTEN-FREE CRACKERS AND RICE CAKES: Hol-Grain onion and garlic brown rice gluten-free crackers; Real Foods and Lundberg Family Farms brands brown rice cakes.

GUT FLUSH TIP • Check out www.glutenfreemall.com for these products and others.

GLUTEN-FREE HOT AND COLD CEREALS: Various brands of unsweetened cereals, such as Nu-World puffed amaranth, Arrowhead Mills amaranth, and Rice & Shine cream of rice cereals, Ancient Harvest quinoa flakes, Bob's Red Mill creamy rice hot cereal, and Lundberg Family Farms Hot 'n Creamy rice cereal, Arrowhead Mills or Lundberg Family Farms oats, Earth Song Grandpa's Secret Omega-3 muesli.

GUT FLUSH TIP • Many of these cereals may be unfamiliar to you. It is my hope once you become accustomed to their natural goodness, you won't want to go back to eating that "sugary stuff" again. Experiment with the various tastes and textures and see which ones will become your favorites.

COOKING AND BAKING PRODUCTS: Salt (Morton's canning and pickling salt, Celtic sea salt); aluminum-free baking powder (Rumford, Royal, Featherweight, Ener-G); thickeners (Eden kuzu and arrowroot); tapioca; coconut (Frontier shredded coconut); alcohol-free vanilla, anise, lemon, and almond extracts (Frontier and Simply Organic); gluten-free flour (Montina gluten-free flour and Montina baking supplement); brown rice, millet, buckwheat, teff, garbanzo, and quinoa flours (Bob's Red Mill) and almond meal.

GUT FLUSH TIP • Those who are extremely gluten intolerant may want to avoid baking soda and baking powder.

OTHER CONDIMENTS: Unfiltered apple cider vinegar (Bragg organic apple cider vinegar), Dijon mustard, coconut milk (Thai Kitchen organic lite coconut milk), lemon and lime juice (Santa Cruz organic lemon and lime juices).

GUT FLUSH TIP • All of the above should be stored in the refrigerator or freezer after opening. Those who are extremely gluten intolerant may want to avoid Dijon mustard.

CANNED INGREDIENTS: Tuna (Natural Sea, Crown Prince), wild salmon (Natural Sea, Crown Prince, Vital Choice), sardines packed in olive oil (Bela, Olhão, Crown Prince), artichoke hearts, capers and hearts of palm (Napoleon, Native Forest), black and green olives (Santa Barbara Co.), organic canned tomato products (Muir Glen, BioNaturae, Eden, Woodstock Farms unsweetened), unsweetened pumpkin and sweet potato puree (Farmers Market pumpkin puree and sweet potato puree).

GUT FLUSH TIP • For meals that are never boring, keep a variety of these canned staples in your pantry at all times.

DRIED BEANS: Lentils, black, adzuki, garbanzo, kidney.

GUT FLUSH TIP • To preserve freshness and keep microbes away, store all dried legumes in the freezer.

WHEY PROTEIN POWDERS: Hormone-free, unheated, non-denatured, lactose-free with no added sugars or artificial sweeteners like aspartame, sucralose, or Splenda (Fat Flush vanilla or chocolate whey protein powder—see Resources).

GUT FLUSH TIP • Whey protein powder is versatile. Try using whey protein powder in your favorite pancake recipe and in baked products such as bread and muffins. Experiment with different smoothie flavors for an exciting taste sensation.

TEAS: African honeybush, Alvita, or traditional medicinal Pau d'Arco (Taheebo), dandelion root, mugwort (bulk), Eden twig tea, chicory root (bulk).

GUT FLUSH TIP • Keep a variety of these teas in your pantry, as each one has unique cleansing properties.

MISCELLANEOUS: Nature's Way slippery elm bark capsules, bulk slippery elm bark, Frontier kelp powder.

GUT FLUSH TIP • Slippery elm tea is a time-honored treatment for indigestion. Keep these capsules in your Gut Flush arsenal.

Establish a Good Water Source

As you know, water is a big part of the Gut Flush Plan. But how do you make sure you're actually getting clean, parasite-free water? The answer is, filter your own. Not only is it way more environmentally friendly than purchasing

THE GUT FLUSH STAPLES SHOPPING LIST

■

I've created this shopping time-saver to help you stock up before you begin the Gut Flush Plan. It includes the grocery staples for all three weeks, compiled into one handy list. Photocopy these pages and take the list with you on your first Gut Flush shopping trip. **Note:** Shopping lists for perishable foods are located after each week's meal plan.

Equipment:

Meat thermometer

Oil sprayer (like the Misto)

Vegetable steamer (optional)

Parchment paper

Dried Herbs and Spices

(1 small bottle of each)
Look for organic nonirradiated dried herbs and spices without additives.

Basil

Bay leaves

Cardamom

Cayenne pepper

Celery seed

Cinnamon

Cloves (ground)

Coriander

Cumin (ground)

Curry powder

Dill

Fennel seeds (can buy ground)

Garlic powder

Ginger

Gomasio (sesame salt)

Italian seasoning

Marjoram

Mustard, dry

Nutmeg, ground

Oregano

Poultry seasoning

Red pepper flakes

Rosemary (can buy ground)

Sage

Thyme

Turmeric

Oils

Coconut oil (unrefined)	12-oz jar
Fish oil (lemon-flavored)	12-oz bottle
Flaxseed oil	16-oz bottle
Olive oil	16-oz bottle
Sesame oil	8-oz bottle

Nuts and Seeds

Flaxseed (ground)	24 oz
Pumpkin seeds (shelled)	½ lb
Sesame seeds	¼ lb
Sunflower seeds (shelled)	¾ lb
Almond butter (unsweetened)	1 small jar
Tahini (sesame seed butter)	1 small jar
Almonds	1 lb
Brazil nuts	½ lb
Pine nuts	¾ lb
Walnuts	1½ lb

Grocery

Almond milk	1 qt
Apple cider vinegar (unfiltered)	16-oz bottle
Artichoke hearts (packed in water)	2 14-oz cans
Baking powder (nonaluminum)	1 small can
Baking soda	1 small box
Broth, beef	3 32-oz boxes
Broth, chicken	32-oz box
Broth, vegetable	2 32-oz boxes
Capers	1 small bottle
Coconut milk (unsweetened)	14-oz can
Dijon mustard	1 small bottle
Marinara sauce	2 15-oz jars
Tomato paste	6-oz can
Tomatoes, crushed	2 14-oz cans
Tomatoes, diced	2 14-oz cans
Salmon, wild	4 7-oz cans
Salt	1 box
Sardines (olive oil–packed, with bones)	2 4-oz packages
Tuna (light water-packed)	2 7-oz cans
Vanilla extract	1 small bottle
Water (filtered or purified)	3 qt
	(not including amount needed for drinking water and making tea)

Grains, Flours, Pasta, and Dried Beans

Amaranth, unsweetened puffed cereal	1 small box
Buckwheat	¼ lb
Gluten-free flour (Montina)	1 small package
Millet	1 lb
Oats	1 lb
Quinoa	1 lb
Quinoa flakes	1 small box
Quinoa flour	½ lb

Rice (brown or wild)	1 lb
Pasta, rice	½ lb
Pasta, whole soybean	½ lb
Beans, black	½ lb
Beans, garbanzo	½ lb

Frozen

Blueberries	10-oz bag
Raspberries	10-oz bag
Strawberries	10-oz bag
Spinach	10-oz box
Rice pecan bread	1 loaf
Turkey burgers (100% turkey)	1 box (or can use fresh ground turkey)
Turkey sausage patties	1 box

Refrigerated

Butter	½ lb
Sauerkraut, raw	16-oz jar
Vegenaise	1 small jar
Yellow miso	1 small container

Gut Flush Plan Essentials

Roasted chicory root tea (bulk only), dandelion root, African honeybush tea (*one or more*)	1 box (for Week One)
Pau d'Arco and/or mugwort tea	1 box (for Week Two)
Slippery elm capsules	1 bottle (for Week Three)
Kelp powder	1 small bottle
Fat Flush vanilla whey (Uni Key)	2-lb jar
Flora-Key (Uni Key)	5-oz jar

large quantities of bottled water, but as we've discussed previously, the fact that your water is bottled is in no way a guarantee of purity.

One of my favorite products is the Doulton ceramic water filter, which has pores tiny enough to remove parasites, bacteria, and particles as small as 0.5 microns. A great thing about this filter is that it works in three stages. First, the little pores take out the pathogens, dirt, and rust. Then the filter eliminates pesticides, chlorine, and chemicals. The final stage removes heavy metals. The filter is both efficient and long-lasting. If you have a family of four, you won't have to change the filter more than once a year.

If you absolutely must buy your water, get it in glass or ceramic containers. Plastic containers can leach chemicals into the water.

When using tap water, only use the cold for cooking or drinking. The hot water has a greater risk of containing stuff like lead, asbestos, and other contaminants. And don't forget to run the cold water for a minute or two before using, or lead leached from the pipes may get into your water. Better yet, have a water filter installed under your sink, so you don't have to worry about the purity of what's coming out of the tap.

Because water is a large contributor to parasitical infections, I recommend that you take steps to make sure the water that enters your home is as safe as possible. Check the safety record of your local water company (go to www.epa.gov/OGWDW/dwinfo.htm for more information) or call the EPA to test your tap water (800-426-4791 or, if you live in Washington, D.C., or Alaska, 202-382-5533).

Create Your Gut Flush Food Journal

The last step in your preparation for the Gut Flush Plan is the creation of your own Gut Flush Food Journal. Multiple studies have shown that people are way more likely to adhere to their planned food programs when they use a food journal.

As you probably already know from personal experience, a giant factor in bad food habits is stress. But experts note that journaling can often help you defang that stress as well as help you plot strategies to avoid bad food habits in the future. When you are tempted to indulge in food that you would never eat during a calmer mood, a brief session of noting your emotions in your food journal may help you head off that binge. That's why I recommend incorporating information on your emotions and your motivations in your journal.

When you review your food journal at the end of each week, you'll be able to look back and see your "triggers," situations that might cause you to eat in a way that's not in your best interests. When you actually write down what's going on in your life and note how your diet corresponds to those events, you can tamp down your food-related anxieties and take a big step toward resolving personal issues that have hampered your health.

One thing: You *must* be honest in your journal and don't hold back. That's the only way to make your journal an effective tool to aid you in resolving your Gut Flush issues. Make notes about your emotions, your hunger, your cravings, and your physical symptoms (cramps, stomach pain, nausea, diarrhea, etc.) so that when you review your journal you can take concrete steps to avoid these problems.

By tracking your physical responses to foods, you can more easily identify which foods are causing your problems. Even if you don't follow the Gut Flush Plan verbatim, the food journal can help you zero in on trouble areas: Do you get nauseated every time you down a milk product? Are you in a consistent fog after eating bread? Do you have a sleepless night after three cups of coffee in the afternoon? A journal helps to make these patterns evident.

Don't be overly critical of yourself in your journal. You want the experiences to be a positive one that helps you grow. Yes, you want to recognize where your diet may be going off course. But give yourself a break at the same time and realize that the best diet wasn't constructed in a day, a week, or even a month. It may take time to change ingrained habits that you've had for years.

It doesn't matter where you keep your journal as long as it is compiled in a place where you can create consistent entries. If that means using a notebook, index cards, a computer file, or a calendar—whatever works for you— is fine.

Note these categories in your journal:

* What foods you eat and when and where you eat them. Include all meals, snacks, beverages—anything that crosses your lips.

- How you felt before, during, and after eating. What were your emotions and your physical feelings? These indications may be related to your immune response to foods, allergens, and nutrients.
- What supplements are you taking that day? How did they change the way you felt?
- What are the physical problems you want to alleviate and what progress are you feeling in encouraging their departure? For example, if you always have afternoon headaches, note if their intensity has changed, how they correlate with your foods, and what foods you think are most problematic.
- What exercise do you engage in? How does it make you feel? Do you have any aches or pains to worry about?
- Your sleep habits: What time did you go to bed? How long did it take you to fall asleep? How did you feel when you woke up? Did you awaken during the night?
- Other health notes: Is your menstruation normal? Do you have easy bowel movements? Diarrhea? How are your moods and nerves? Are you calm or anxious much of the time? Do these mood swings correspond to foods you eat? Are you having regular sex?
- Use some space in your journal to reflect on how you feel about your life and the addition of the Gut Flush Plan. Are you reaching your life goals? Do these goals need to be adjusted? How do your friends and family members relate to your changes in health habits? Do they encourage or discourage you?

In general, use your journal to establish an overall view of how your Gut Flush Plan is developing. Each night, review your notes for that day; at the end of each week, read back over the past seven days. This can be an incredibly enlightening way to recognize long-term trends in your health and diet. If you make significant progress, reading your journal can also be immensely rewarding. Take time to celebrate the changes you've made and how wonderful they make you feel.

Your journal can help you visualize exactly where you are in your Gut Flush improvements, and what you still must do to move ahead. Creating this mental image of your status and goals will help you stay committed and truly appreciate all the changes, small and large, that the Gut Flush brings to your life.

Right now, before you go any further, write down four goals for the Gut Flush Plan. You might say, "Eliminate my craving for sugar" or "Get rid of these infernal yeast infections." Paste them into the front of your food journal. You might even post them in a place you'll see them every day, like the fridge door.

Now you are truly prepared to begin the Gut Flush Plan, to eradicate the Colon Corruptors, strengthen your GI Good Guys, and revitalize your health, inside and out. Let's get started with the first week of your 21-Day Gut Flush Plan.

11

Week One:
Focus on Fortifying

You've read all the frightening statistics. You know what's at stake in our Food Fright environment. Now it's time to implement the changes that will keep you and your family safe against all Colon Corruptors, both now and in the future. It's time to start the Gut Flush Menu Plan.

By now you know that Gut Flushing is an ongoing process. It doesn't happen overnight. It's not just about following a diet or supplement regimen. It's all about a brand-new lifestyle and looking at foods, your habits, and your environment from a whole different perspective that will keep you healthy for a very long time.

Some of you may have gained dramatic relief already. If you identified a food sensitivity and have eliminated common trouble foods such as wheat and milk, you are probably on the way to relief from symptoms such as constipation, diarrhea, bloat, lack of energy, canker sores, or headaches. Others with more serious disorders such as duodenal ulcers, GERD, irritable bowel syndrome, or Crohn's disease may have found that by introducing a probiotic into your regimen, there has been a marked improvement in your overall health. Perhaps by identifying yeasts and parasites as your particular "hidden invaders," symptoms like skin problems, arthritic-like aches and pains, insomnia, and even depression have done a vanishing act.

Now you are ready for the true "clean sweep." The entire 21-Day Gut Flush Plan is designed to get your digestive system and your whole body humming with vitality, energy, and visible health. The menu plan will help everyone, no matter what their particular health situation, experience the benefits of a Gut Flush. Not only will this program help to root out any of the lingering foods or beverages that might encourage Colon Corruptors, but it is also packed with so many delicious GI-friendly foods that your digestive system and your taste buds will be in heaven.

Each week of the eating program will focus on one of the three steps of the Gut Flush Plan. The main dietary goal in Week One is to help Fortify your entire digestive system by eating satisfying meals full of foods and beverages that bolster your GI Good Guys. You'll eat a diet specifically formulated to recolonize your probiotic population, increase your level of HCl, and encourage the activity of your digestive enzymes. Wholesome proteins, lots of colorful vegetables, and gluten-free grains and starches are all delectably highlighted in the menus.

You'll find a shopping list of the perishable items necessary for Week One at the end of the menu section. Each day of the menus will follow the six important strategies to Fortify your gut that we talked about in Chapter 7.

1. **Single out all remaining sweets, molds, and starches.** For the initial two weeks of the 21-day plan you will not use sugar or artificial sweeteners in any form. That means fruits, fruit juice, sugar alcohols (including xylitol), and even natural sweeteners like honey, maple syrup, agave, and stevia.

2. **Power up on prebiotics and probiotics.** Include at least *two* prebiotics (choose a variety from onions, garlic, Jerusalem artichokes, leeks, asparagus, shallots, jicama, and oregano) and *one* probiotic food daily (think one cup of plain yogurt or kefir, half cup of sauerkraut, or one cup of plain miso).

3. **Fill up on soluble fiber, the fuel that friendly flora in your colon ferment into healing compounds that strengthen your gut.** On a daily

basis, choose at least *two* food sources that are rich in soluble fiber, like oatmeal, vegetables, seeds, nuts, and at least one to two tablespoons of ground flaxseed. (For those with sensitive digestion, please grind your nuts and seeds to a fine powder, and favor steamed or lightly cooked vegetables as opposed to raw.)

4. **Omega-size!** Eat at least four ounces of omega-3-rich fatty fish (salmon, tuna, mackerel, sardines) *twice* a week. Enjoy omega-3 nuts like walnuts and Brazil nuts on salads or as snacks. Incorporate at least one tablespoon *each* of fish oil and flaxseed oil daily in nonheated recipes. Also, on Week One of the 21-Day Gut Flush Plan, you may enjoy up to one tablespoon of olive oil daily (high in the nonessential but healthy omega 9–rich fatty acids) in cooking.

5. **Drink to your health.** Between meals, try to consume at least half of your body weight in ounces of water per day. Add at least two cups per day of a fortifying beverage, like roasted chicory root tea, a coffee substitute such as dandelion root tea, or caffeine-free organic African honeybush tea.

6. **Shake that salt shaker.** If you don't have a medical condition that makes salt less advisable for you (such as high blood pressure, heart problems, or ulcer difficulties), please aim for at least one teaspoon per day spread throughout your meals and snacks.

Dig in and enjoy!

Sample Menu Plans for Week One

Note: Menu items designated with an asterisk (*) appear in the recipe section located in the Appendix, page 227.

DAY 1

BREAKFAST	½ cup cooked oatmeal mixed with 1 tablespoon *each* ground flaxseed and ground almonds ½ cup **Ann Louise's Yogurt*** or plain whole-milk yogurt *(Use a teaspoon of **Flora-Key** for sweetener, if you like.)*
MIDMORNING SNACK	1 cup steamed mixed bell pepper and jicama strips with **Ann Louise's Tangy Tapenade***
LUNCH	*Rainbow Salad* 4 oz grilled chicken mixed with 3 cups steamed arugula and spinach, 4 artichoke hearts ¼ cup *each* radishes and green onions, 2 tablespoons *each* chopped parsley and broccoli sprouts, and 1 tablespoon lemon-flavored fish oil, and sprinkle with 2 tablespoons toasted sunflower seeds
MIDAFTERNOON SNACK	2 hard-boiled eggs with a dash of salt 2 celery stalks topped with 2 teaspoons almond butter mixed with 1 tablespoon ground flaxseed
DINNER	4 oz grilled wild salmon (rubbed with garlic and turmeric before cooking) drizzled with 1 teaspoon olive oil and a squeeze of lime and sprinkled with 1 teaspoon chopped fresh dill 1 cup steamed asparagus sprinkled with salt to taste ½ cup baked butternut squash with cinnamon

Tip of the Day: *Ground flaxseed can be used in a number of ways, including breading for chicken or fish, sprinkled over eggs or salad, and mixed in baked products such as muffins, pancakes, or meat loaf. Flaxseed is a terrific source of soluble fiber, providing 6 grams per one-quarter cup.*

DAY 2

BREAKFAST	2 scrambled eggs (cooked in 2 teaspoons butter and a dash of salt) with ¼ cup *each* chopped onion and bell pepper topped with 1 tablespoon *each* chopped cilantro, salsa, and plain yogurt
MIDMORNING SNACK	1 cup *Ann Louise's Yogurt** or plain whole-milk yogurt mixed with ¼ cup almonds, 1 tablespoon ground flaxseed, and a dash each ground cinnamon, ginger, and cloves *(Use a teaspoon of Flora-Key for sweetener, if you like.)*
LUNCH	4 oz grilled or broiled chicken breast (rubbed with garlic and marjoram prior to cooking) 2 cups *Quick and Easy Carrot Soup** topped with 1 tablespoon toasted pumpkin seeds Salad of mixed greens, tomato, cucumber, and green onions tossed with 2 tablespoons *Lemon Caper Dressing**
MIDAFTERNOON SNACK	½ avocado stuffed with ¼ cup water-packed tuna, mixed with 2 teaspoons Vegenaise, squeeze of lemon, and 1 tablespoon *each* chopped cilantro and broccoli sprouts
DINNER	1 serving *Turkey Meat Loaf Florentine** ½ cup steamed brown rice mixed with 1 tablespoon chopped walnuts, a dash of salt, ¼ teaspoon dried oregano, and cayenne to taste 2 cups steamed baby bok choy drizzled with 1 tablespoon lemon-flavored fish oil

Tip of the Day: Yes, avocados are one of the good fats. They also have 60 percent more potassium than bananas, as well as vitamins B, E, and K. Don't forget they're a good source of soluble fiber, too. One half of an avocado provides 2 grams of soluble fiber and is soothing to the entire digestive tract.

DAY 3

BREAKFAST	1 cup cooked quinoa flakes mixed with ½ cup plain kefir, 1 tablespoon ground flaxseed, and a dash *each* ground nutmeg, cinnamon, and ginger *(Use a teaspoon of Flora-Key for sweetener, if you like.)*
MIDMORNING SNACK	1 cup *Miso Soup Plus** 1 cup steamed cauliflower and broccoli florets
LUNCH	1 serving last night's *Turkey Meat Loaf Florentine** on a bed of 2 cups steamed baby spinach ½ cup *each* cherry tomatoes and sliced carrots 1 tablespoon *each* chopped green onions and dill, tossed with 1 tablespoon lemon-flavored fish oil and 1½ teaspoons apple cider vinegar sprinkled with sesame seeds or gomasio (sesame salt)
MIDAFTERNOON SNACK	1 cup cucumber and radish slices, ½ cup *Ann Louise's Yogurt** or plain whole-milk yogurt mixed with 1 tablespoon chopped walnuts, ⅛ teaspoon ground ginger, and cayenne to taste
DINNER	3 cups *Savory Turkey and Swiss Chard Soup** 1 cup *each* steamed yellow squash and asparagus with 2 tablespoons *each* red onion and chopped fresh dill drizzled with 1 tablespoon *Lemon Caper Dressing** and sprinkled with 1 tablespoon ground flaxseed

Tip of the Day: Food safety is absolutely an underrated and ignored key to good health, particularly digestive health. Refrigerate leftovers (such as the **Turkey Meat Loaf Florentine**) immediately after the meal to ensure harmful bacteria do not grow on your food. This timely storage does not harm the refrigerator's operation.

BREAKFAST	2 "fried" eggs (cooked in 2 teaspoons butter and dash salt) placed on a bed of 2 cups steamed kale and drizzled with 1 tablespoon lemon-flavored fish oil 1 cup plain kefir mixed with ¼ cup chopped walnuts, a dash of ground cinnamon, and 1 tablespoon ground flaxseed *(Use a teaspoon of Flora-Key for sweetener if you like.)*
MIDMORNING SNACK	1 cup beef broth with 2 tablespoons chopped green onions
LUNCH	4 oz sardines (canned) wrapped in romaine leaves and topped with grated jicama, onions, and broccoli florets
MIDAFTERNOON SNACK	1 cup *each* steamed zucchini and snow peas ½ cup **Ann Louise's Yogurt*** or plain whole-milk yogurt mixed with 1 teaspoon *each* ground cumin and chopped cilantro and 1 tablespoon ground flaxseed
DINNER	1 cup cooked whole soybean pasta tossed with 1 cup *each* steamed chopped broccoli and red bell pepper, ½ cup marinara sauce, red pepper flakes and salt to taste, 2 tablespoons chopped shallots, and ½ teaspoon fennel seed, and topped with 1 tablespoon toasted pine nuts 2 cups endive, ½ cup chopped Jerusalem artichokes, and 2 tablespoons *each* shredded beets and carrots tossed with 1 tablespoon **Lemon Caper Dressing***

Tip of the Day: *Today's dinner includes the Jerusalem artichoke, or sunchoke as it is sometimes called. This nutty vegetable is a small tuber similar to a potato without the high carbohydrate level. This "artichoke" is loaded with iron, potassium, and thiamine, and is another good source of the prebiotic inulin.*

DAY 5

BREAKFAST	2 turkey sausage patties on a bed of 1 cup steamed fennel, topped with 2 tablespoons chopped walnuts
MIDMORNING SNACK	5 baby carrots and ½ cup jicama sticks 1 tablespoon *each* almond butter and ground flaxseed
LUNCH	*Salmon and Asparagus* 4 oz wild salmon (canned) mixed with 1 tablespoon *each* chopped cilantro and parsley, and ¼ cup *each* chopped celery, radish, and green onions, and tossed with 1 tablespoon flaxseed oil and juice of ½ lime 1 cup steamed asparagus topped with 2 tablespoons chopped Brazil nuts
MIDAFTERNOON SNACK	2 chopped hard-boiled eggs mixed with a dash of dry mustard, 1 tablespoon *each* chopped red onion and fresh dill, 1 tablespoon lemon-flavored fish oil, and 1 tablespoon ground flaxseed
DINNER	4 oz lean ground beef burger topped with ½ cup *Simple Homemade Sauerkraut** (or from a jar) ¼ cup broccoli sprouts 1 small roasted yam sprinkled with ground cinnamon, ginger, turmeric, a dash of salt, and 1 tablespoon toasted pumpkin seeds ½ cup *each* sliced onion and sugar snap peas sautéed in 1 tablespoon olive oil, 2 teaspoons chopped garlic, and a dash of salt, and topped with 1 tablespoon chopped fresh oregano

Tip of the Day: Sauerkraut, one of our premier probiotic foods, is also an excellent source of vitamin C and contains more lactobacilli than yogurt. Sauerkraut can also be eaten cold with lemon, oil, and green onions as a salad.

DAY 6

BREAKFAST	½ cup cooked millet mixed with 1 tablespoon *each* chopped walnuts and ground flaxseed ½ cup *Ann Louise's Yogurt** or plain whole-milk yogurt *(Use a teaspoon of Flora-Key for sweetener, if you like.)*
MIDMORNING SNACK	½ cup *each* broccoli florets and carrot sticks with ¼ cup *Ann Louise's Tangy Tapenade**
LUNCH	*Tomato Stuffed with Tuna* 4 oz tuna (canned) mixed with 2 teaspoons *each* chopped green olives and almonds 2 tablespoons *each* chopped celery and bell pepper, and ¼ teaspoon dried oregano and salt to taste, tossed with 1 tablespoon flaxseed oil and juice of ½ lemon and stuffed into a hollowed-out tomato
MIDAFTERNOON SNACK	1 cup *Miso Soup Plus** sprinkled with 1 tablespoon ground flaxseed
DINNER	4 oz *Amaranth and Herb-Crusted Chicken** 1 cup grilled yellow squash salted to taste 1 cup steamed kale drizzled with 1 tablespoon lemon-flavored fish oil and topped with 1 teaspoon *each* chopped garlic and fennel seeds

Tip of the Day: Although purslane is a succulent green leafy vegetable commonly eaten in Greece, many Americans have never heard of it. The plant's leaves are high in omega-3s, as well as a rich plant source of melatonin. You can grow this treasure chest of nutrients to add to your soups and your favorite cucumber and yogurt dishes. It can even serve as healthy substitute for the steamed kale on tonight's menu.

HOW TO STEAM AN ARTICHOKE

Cut off about 1 inch from top and bottom. Add 1 inch water to a steamer; place artichoke into pan, stem down. Cover; cook 25 to 40 minutes, or until leaves can easily be removed.

DAY 7

BREAKFAST	2-egg omelet (cooked in 2 teaspoons butter and a dash of salt) with ¼ cup *each* chopped bell pepper and baby spinach, 2 teaspoons *each* chopped shallot and olives, sprinkled with dried basil and oregano and topped with 1 tablespoon salsa
MIDMORNING SNACK	1 cup mixture steamed snow peas and baby carrots 1 tablespoon almond butter
LUNCH	4 oz grilled or pan-fried turkey burger ½ cup *each* sliced red onion and zucchini sautéed in 1 tablespoon olive oil and topped with 2 teaspoons Dijon mustard, sliced tomatoes, ¼ cup clover sprouts, and 1 tablespoon chopped parsley
MIDAFTERNOON SNACK	1 cup ***Ann Louise's Yogurt*** or plain whole-milk yogurt mixed with a dash *each* ground cinnamon, nutmeg, and ginger, 1 tablespoon ground flaxseed, and ¼ cup chopped walnuts *(Use a teaspoon of Flora-Key for sweetener if you like.)*
DINNER	4 oz grilled salmon with ***Parsley and Cilantro Pesto**** Steamed artichoke drizzled with 1 tablespoon lemon-flavored fish oil 2 cups mixed greens (mustard, kale, collards) braised in ¼ cup chicken stock with ⅛ teaspoon ground fennel seed and sprinkled with ¼ teaspoon *each* caraway and sesame seeds

Tip of the Day: *Did you know that flaxseed can be used in tea to soothe your tummy and GI tract? Steep one teaspoon ground flaxseed in eight ounces boiling water for twenty minutes; strain. Drink one cup per day in addition to your other* Fortifying *beverages.*

Week One Perishables Shopping List

This list includes all the perishables for Week One of the Gut Flush Plan. (Note: The staples shopping list is located in Chapter 10, "Getting Ready for Gut Flush.")

Produce

Lemons	About 8 (or as needed)
Limes	2 to 4 (or as needed)
Artichoke, globe	1 medium
Asparagus	1 pound
Avocado	1 medium
Beets	1 small bunch
Bell pepper, green	2
Bell pepper, orange	2
Bell pepper, red	2
Bok choy, baby	1
Broccoli	1 head
Broccoli sprouts	1 package
Brussels sprouts	1½ lb
Cabbage, green	1 medium head
Carrots, baby	1 small bag
Carrots, large	1 bunch or 1-lb bag
Cauliflower	1 small head
Celery	1 bunch
Cucumber	1 large
Garlic	3 heads
Ginger	1 small head
Greens, arugula	1 small head
Greens, collards	1 small bunch
Greens, endive	1 small bunch
Greens, fennel	1 small bunch
Greens, kale	1 small bunch
Greens, mustard	1 small bunch

Greens, romaine (or other lettuce)	1 head
Greens, salad	3-oz package
Greens, Swiss chard	1 small bunch
Jerusalem artichoke	1 medium
Jicama	1 large
Onion, green	1 bunch
Onion, red	1
Onion, white or yellow	3 medium
Radish	1 bunch
Radish, daikon	1 small
Shallots	3–4
Snow pea pods	½ lb
Spinach, baby	2 3-oz bags or 1 5-oz container
Squash, butternut	1 medium
Squash, yellow	2 medium
Squash, zucchini	1 medium
Sugar snap peas	½ lb
Sweet potato (optional)	1 small
Tomatoes	2 medium
Tomatoes, cherry	½ pint
Yam	1 small
Basil	1 bunch
Chives	1 small bunch
Cilantro	1 bunch
Dill	1 small bunch
Oregano	1 bunch
Parsley	1 to 2 bunches
Thyme	1 small bunch

Dairy

Milk (whole or 2%)	2 quarts *(needed if making own yogurt)*
Yogurt, unsweetened, plain (whole or low-fat)	2 quarts *(needed if NOT making own yogurt)*

Lean Protein

Eggs	1 dozen
Ground beef	6 oz
Boneless, skinless chicken breast	8 5-oz breasts
Boneless, skinless turkey breast	1¼ lb
Ground turkey	1 lb (1¼ lb breast, 6-oz thigh if possible)
Salmon fillet	2 4-oz (4 oz each for days 1 and 7)

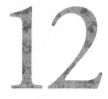

Week Two:
Focus on Flushing

WEEK TWO OF THE 21-DAY GUT FLUSH PLAN CONTINUES THE MOMEN-
tum begun in Week One. This week we'll flush out any remaining parasites,
yeast, food sensitivities, and Superbugs. You will continue to enjoy many of
the wonderful foods outlined in Week One, including the high-fiber and pre-
biotic- and probiotic-based foods and supplements. I invite you to continue
with your digestive aids as well.

For this week, if you have not already, I would encourage you to add a
high-fiber supplement to the program, especially if constipation is still a challenge. Moving your bowels at least once or twice daily is the goal. Regarding
a natural laxative, the Super-GI Cleanse (see Resources) would be my personal choice because this product contains gentle herbs that help to enhance
the flushing process by removing parasites (butternut root bark), soothing the
irritated mucous membranes of the digestive tract (licorice root), and relieving gas (peppermint leaves).

For those with loose stools or diarrhea, the continued use of the probiotics will be key, but a high-fiber supplement like Super-GI Cleanse
should be avoided for now. In the case of continuing diarrhea, the use of the
L-glutamine supplements suggested in Step 3: Feed, on page 127, might be

very helpful, with a dose of 500–1,000 mg about twenty minutes before meals three times daily. L-glutamine, among its other claims to fame, "firms up" the bowel.

If you are focusing on parasites and yeast, at this time you may wish to integrate the Para-Key, Verma-Plus, and Flora-Key formulas from My Colon Cleansing Kit or similar products. (See chapters 3 and 4 for specific protocol suggestions.) Also, if yeast is your target, then consider introducing the Y-C Cleanse (see Resources) upon arising, perhaps fifteen to twenty minutes in the morning before you take your probiotics. Including a product containing Saccharomyces boulardii (a friendly yeast) with the probiotics in the a.m. and p.m. will help to further support gastrointestinal health. (My favorite brand is Thornes Sacro-B (see Resources). This nonpathogenic yeast supplement is both very supportive for people with inflammatory bowel disease and a specific help during or following antibiotic therapy, especially if you have a C. difficile (antibiotic-induced) infection.

You'll find a perishables shopping list for Week Two immediately following the menu plans. This week's meal plan will focus on the six Flushing strategies we discussed in Chapter 8:

1. **Bet on beta-carotene.** I would like you to enjoy at least *two servings* of beta-carotene–rich foods every day.
2. **Go *coconutty!*** This week, as in Week One, you'll also continue to take *one tablespoon each of flaxseed and fish oil* every day, to support your cellular membranes. Instead of Week One's olive oil, however, I would like you to use *one tablespoon of coconut oil* several times a week.
3. **Keep out the unfriendly carbs.** Enjoy up to *two* servings daily of gluten-free grains and starches such as quinoa, buckwheat, amaranth, brown rice, and millet. Please note you will continue to avoid all fruit and fruit juices as well as all other sweeteners until Week Three.
4. **Spice up your life.** During Week Two, you will find oregano and cinnamon on the menu several times a week and both garlic and cayenne used on a daily basis.
5. **Add more Colon Corruptor killer foods to your diet.** Include at least one-quarter to one-half cup ground or whole pumpkin seeds, a dash of

kelp granules on your veggies, one-half cup sauerkraut, a handful of al-monds, and at least a radish a day.

6. **Add Flushing beverages to your day.** In addition to continuing to drink-ing *half your body weight in ounces* of water, add at least *two* cups of a Flushing beverage. (This drink will take the place of Week One's Fortify-ing beverages.) Choose from Pau d'Arco (also known as Taheebo) and/or mugwort tea.

Sample Menu Plans for Week Two

DAY 1

BREAKFAST	½ cup toasted oats (brown in dry pan over medium heat in 1 tablespoon coconut oil) mixed into ½ cup unsweetened almond milk with 1 tablespoon *each* ground flaxseed and chopped walnuts *(Use a teaspoon of Flora-Key for sweetener, if you like.)*
MIDMORNING SNACK	½ cup lightly steamed mixed vegetables ¼ cup **Ann Louise's Tangy Tapenade***
LUNCH	*Sardine Salad* 4 oz can sardines packed in olive oil on bed of 2 cups torn or shredded romaine lettuce with ¼ cup *each* sliced radishes, celery, cucumber, and bell pepper, drizzled with 1 tablespoon lemon-flavored fish oil and juice of ½ lime 1 **Almond Meal Muffin***
MIDAFTERNOON SNACK	½ cup **Simple Homemade Sauerkraut** (or from a jar) mixed with ¼ cup toasted pumpkin seeds *(Use a teaspoon of Flora-Key for sweetener, if you like.)*
DINNER	6 oz oven-roasted lamb chop (rubbed with dry mustard, garlic, and cumin before cooking) ¼ cup raw long-grain brown rice cooked in ½ cup vegetable broth and 2 teaspoons minced garlic, mixed with 2 tablespoons chopped green onions (¼ cup raw rice = ½ cup cooked) 2 cups steamed collards (or greens of your choice) with ½ cup *each* steamed julienne carrots and yellow peppers, tossed with 1 tablespoon *each* flaxseed oil and lemon juice, 1 teaspoon *each* chopped garlic, oregano, and parsley, and a dash *each* salt and kelp granules

Tip of the Day: Heavy intake of raw vegetables as well as very cold or iced drinks and foods should be curtailed. These foods cause the intestines to contract, thereby holding in toxins rather than releasing them.

DAY 2

BREAKFAST	1 slice *Mega-Grain Quick Bread** drizzled with 1 tablespoon flaxseed oil 1 cup plain kefir mixed with 1 tablespoon ground almonds and a dash *each* ground cloves, cinnamon, and ginger *(Use a teaspoon of Flora-Key for sweetener, if you like.)*
MIDMORNING SNACK	½ cup warm artichoke hearts and 5 black olives with a splash of lemon and sprinkle of chopped dill
LUNCH	*Chopped Salad* 4 oz wild salmon (canned) mixed with 1 cup *each* chopped green and red cabbage, ½ cup *each* bean sprouts and chopped red bell pepper, and 2 tablespoons *each* chopped daikon radish and red onion, tossed with 1 tablespoon lemon-flavored fish oil and ½ teaspoon *each* chopped thyme and garlic, and sprinkled with kelp granules
MIDAFTERNOON SNACK	1 cup chicken broth with ¼ cup cooked brown rice, 1 tablespoon chopped chives, and a dash of cayenne
DINNER	4 oz baked snapper coated with 2 tablespoons ground walnuts, a dash *each* salt and cayenne, and ½ teaspoon *each* dried oregano and ground fennel seed ½ cup cooked quinoa tossed with ¼ teaspoon dried basil and 1 tablespoon *each* coconut oil and ground flaxseed 1 cup Swiss chard braised in 1 cup vegetable broth and 1 teaspoon *each* chopped shallot and garlic sprinkled with gomasio (sesame salt)

Tip of the Day: Almonds are known to have antiparasitic properties and are often found in enzyme combinations that can help digest a variety of uninvited "guests."

DAY 3

BREAKFAST	½ cup cooked oatmeal, mixed with ½ cup plain kefir, 1 tablespoon ground flaxseed and a dash *each* ground nutmeg, cinnamon, and cloves
MIDMORNING SNACK	½ avocado and ½ cup cherry tomatoes drizzled with 1 tablespoon **Lemon Caper Dressing***
LUNCH	**Egg Salad Wraps** 2 chopped hard-boiled eggs mixed with a dash of dry mustard, 2 teaspoons *each* chopped onion, celery, garlic, and radish, and 1 tablespoon lemon-flavored fish oil, divided between 2 steamed red leaf lettuce leaves and folded to form "wraps." ½ cup *each* steamed broccoli and baby carrots sprinkled with 1 tablespoon chopped cilantro and a dash of kelp granules
MIDAFTERNOON SNACK	1 cup **Ann Louise's Yogurt*** or plain whole-milk yogurt mixed with ¼ cup chopped Brazil nuts and a dash of ground cinnamon and ginger *(Use a teaspoon of Flora-Key for sweetener, if you like.)*
DINNER	4 oz grilled chicken (rubbed with garlic and ¼ teaspoon *each* dried oregano and lime juice before cooking) ½ cup steamed sugar snap peas sprinkled with dill 2 cups grilled red peppers and zucchini 1 small baked yam mashed with 1 tablespoon *each* coconut oil and ground pumpkin seeds and a pinch of ground cardamom

Tip of the Day: *Protein foods—meat, fish, eggs, and poultry—supply the amino-acid building blocks needed to enhance immunity and strengthen tissues.*

DAY 4

BREAKFAST	*French Toast* 2 slices *Mega-Grain Quick Bread** dipped in a mixture of 1 egg and 2 tablespoons coconut milk and a dash *each* ground cinnamon and cloves
MIDMORNING SNACK	½ cup *Simple Homemade Sauerkraut* (or from a jar) mixed with ¼ cup *each* chopped bell pepper and carrots, ¼ teaspoon dried oregano, and a dash of cayenne, topped with 1 tablespoon ground almonds and a sprinkling of kelp granules
LUNCH	4 slices organic deli turkey, each wrapped around a cucumber spear *Spinach Salad* 2 cups steamed baby spinach mixed with ½ cup *each* chopped tomato and jicama, 1 tablespoon *each* chopped cilantro and parsley, and 1 tablespoon *each* ground flaxseed and chopped walnuts, tossed with 1 tablespoon lemon-flavored fish oil
MIDAFTERNOON SNACK	1 cup steamed broccoli and red and/or orange bell peppers 1 cup beef broth mixed with 1 tablespoon *each* sliced green onions and radish
DINNER	4 oz pan-seared beef tenderloin (rubbed with garlic and cayenne before cooking) ½ baked acorn squash topped with 1 tablespoon flaxseed oil, ½ teaspoon crushed fennel seed, and a dash of ground cinnamon 2 cups Chinese cabbage steamed with 1 teaspoon *each* sliced garlic and shallots

Tip of the Day: *Raw garlic can be a very effective "natural medicine" that also helps to lower cholesterol. Use it in your recipes every day.*

BREAKFAST	2 eggs poached hard topped with 2 tablespoons *each* sautéed chopped onion and bell pepper and 1 tablespoon *each* chopped basil and oregano, drizzled with 1 tablespoon flaxseed oil 1 cup plain kefir mixed with 1 tablespoon ground flaxseed, and a dash *each* ground cinnamon, cloves, and ginger *(Use a teaspoon of Flora-Key for sweetener, if you like.)*
MIDMORNING SNACK	2 celery stalks 1 tablespoon almond butter
LUNCH	4 oz chicken poached in 2 cups chicken broth with lemon and fresh dill ½ cup baby carrots seasoned with ¼ teaspoon dried sage and a dash each salt and cayenne ½ cup *Simple Homemade Sauerkraut** (or from a jar) drizzled with 1 tablespoon lemon-flavored fish oil
MIDAFTERNOON SNACK	1 cup vegetable broth with 1 tablespoon sliced radish ¼ cup chopped walnuts
DINNER	4 oz firm tofu stir-fried in 2 tablespoons vegetable broth and 1 tablespoon *each* chopped fresh ginger and garlic, sprinkled with kelp granules ½ cup steamed brown rice mixed with 1 tablespoon *each* coconut oil and ground flaxseed and 1 tablespoon toasted pumpkin seeds 2 cups green cabbage braised with a dash of salt ½ cup canned chopped tomatoes, ½ cup sliced red onion, and ½ teaspoon dried oregano

Tip of the Day: Cayenne not only "zings" H. pylori but also is soothing to irritated tissues and helps breaks up congestion.

DAY 6

BREAKFAST	½ cup toasted oats mixed with 1 cup *Ann Louise's Yogurt** or plain whole-milk yogurt, ¼ cup toasted pine nuts, a dash of ground cinnamon, and 1 tablespoon *each* coconut oil and ground flaxseed *(Use a teaspoon of Flora-Key for sweetener, if you like.)*
MIDMORNING SNACK	2 chopped hard-boiled eggs mixed with ¼ cup *each* chopped parsley, radish, and tomatoes, 1 tablespoon *Ranch Dressing** and a dash of cayenne
LUNCH	*Tuna Salad* 4 oz tuna (canned) mixed with ½ cup *each* chopped red cabbage and jicama, ½ cup *each* chopped green onions and celery ¼ cup chopped canned artichoke hearts 1 tablespoon *each* chopped parsley and cilantro, 1 tablespoon flaxseed oil, and juice of ½ lemon
MIDAFTERNOON SNACK	1 cup chicken broth with ¼ cup spinach leaves sprinkled with gomasio (sesame salt) and ¼ cup walnuts
DINNER	4 oz sliced baked turkey breast (season 1 lb turkey breast with ¼ teaspoon *each* dried oregano, basil, thyme, and sage before cooking) 2 cups baby bok choy steamed with 2 teaspoons *each* minced garlic and chopped fresh ginger served over ½ cup cooked millet mixed with 1 tablespoon *each* chopped shallots and radishes and drizzled with 1 tablespoon lemon-flavored fish oil (Cook ½ cup raw millet in 1 cup chicken broth for about 25 minutes. Save remaining millet and turkey breast for tomorrow's soup.)

Tip of the Day: It's particularly important to chew fibrous foods slowly and carefully so these foods can do an efficient job binding up toxins and carrying them through the digestive system.

BREAKFAST	2 turkey sausage patties topped with 1 poached hard egg on bed of 1 cup steamed baby spinach and drizzled with 1 tablespoon *Must-Have Miso Dressing**
MIDMORNING SNACK	1 cup mixture sugar snap peas, radish, and jicama sticks ½ cup *Simple Homemade Sauerkraut** (or from a jar) mixed with 2 tablespoons chopped pumpkin seeds and sprinkled with cayenne
LUNCH	3 cups *Turkey Vegetable Soup* In a medium saucepan, heat 1 cup last night's leftover chopped turkey, ½ cup last night's leftover millet, 2 cups chicken broth, 1 teaspoon minced garlic, ¼ cup *each* chopped carrot, celery, broccoli, onions, and asparagus (or other leftover vegetables), ½ teaspoon *each* dried thyme and oregano, 2 tablespoons *each* chopped parsley and cilantro Simmer about 10 minutes.
MIDAFTERNOON SNACK	1 cup *Ann Louise's Yogurt* or plain whole-milk yogurt mixed with ¼ cup *each* chopped carrot and cucumber and 1 tablespoon *each* ground flaxseed and chopped dill
DINNER	4 oz grilled ground sirloin (rubbed with garlic before cooking) 1 cup *Quinoa Tabbouli** 2 cups steamed mixed collards and kale tossed with 1 tablespoon lemon-flavored fish oil and 1 tablespoon ground flaxseed and a sprinkling of kelp granules

Tip of the Day: Quinoa, an ancient grain dating back to the Inca civilization, is a wonderful gluten-free choice. This protein- and fiber-rich food pairs perfectly with any beef, poultry, and fish meal. Breakfast boredom vanishes when you substitute quinoa for your routine hot cereal.

Week Two Perishables Shopping List

This list includes all the perishables for Week Two of the Gut Flush Plan. (Note: The staples shopping list is located in Chapter 10, "Getting Ready for Gut Flush.")

Produce

Lemons	About 8 (or as needed)
Limes	4 (or as needed)
Asparagus	¼ lb (if none left over from Week One)
Avocado	1 medium
Bean sprouts	1 package
Beets	1 small bunch
Bell pepper, green	1
Bell pepper, orange	2
Bell pepper, red	2
Bell pepper, yellow	1
Bok choy, baby	1 bunch
Broccoli	1 head
Broccoli sprouts	1 package
Cabbage, Chinese	1 small head
Cabbage, green	1 medium head
Cabbage, red	1 medium head
Carrots, baby	1 small bag
Carrots, large	1 bunch or 1-lb bag
Cauliflower	1 small head
Celery	1 bunch
Cucumber	1 large
Garlic	3 heads (or as needed)
Ginger	1 small head
Greens, collards	1 small bunch
Greens, fennel	1 small bunch
Greens, kale	1 small bunch

Greens, romaine (or other lettuce)	1 head
Greens, Swiss chard	1 bunch
Jerusalem artichoke	1 medium
Jicama	1 large
Onion, green	1 bunch
Onion, white or yellow	3 medium
Radish	1 bunch
Radish, daikon	1 small
Shallots	3
Sugar snap peas	½ lb
Spinach, baby	3-oz bag
Squash, acorn	1 medium
Squash, zucchini	2 medium
Tomatoes	2 medium
Tomatoes, cherry	½ pint
Yam	1 small
Basil	1 bunch
Chives	1 small bunch
Cilantro	1 bunch
Dill	1 small bunch
Mint	1 small bunch
Oregano	1 bunch
Parsley	1 bunch

Soy and Dairy

Miso, yellow	1 small container (if needed)
Tofu, firm	1 small container
Kefir, plain unsweetened	1 quart *(for weeks Two and Three)*
Milk (whole or 2%)	2 quarts *(needed if making own yogurt)*
Yogurt, unsweetened, plain (whole or low-fat)	2 quarts *(needed if NOT making own yogurt)*

Lean Protein

Eggs	1 dozen
Deli turkey, sliced (organic, if possible)	2 oz
Lamb chop (bone included)	6 oz
Beef, tenderloin	6 oz
Beef, ground	6 oz
Boneless skinless chicken breast	2 (5 oz each) breasts
Boneless skinless turkey breast	1 lb *(use extra for leftovers)*
Snapper fillet	4 oz

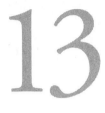

Week Three:
Focus on Feeding

WEEK THREE OF THE 21-DAY GUT FLUSH PLAN REPRESENTS A CULMI-nation of everything you have put into play for the past two weeks. As mentioned in Chapter 9, the menu plan in Week Three is really the model for how I would like you to use the Gut Flush Plan for life.

Of course, you will continue your daily usage of probiotics, HCl, and digestive enzymes. This Gut Flush Basic Protocol should remain a daily habit for life, an essential part of your maintenance routine even after Week Three to ensure future protection from reinfestation of the Colon Corruptors.

Moving into this week and beyond, you may persevere with your protocols for yeast, parasites, Superbugs, and food intolerances until your symptoms disappear. If you are targeting parasites and worms, then by all means continue your parasite-control products during Week Three and thereafter until you complete the timeline for the protocol as discussed in Chapter 4. Many individuals then follow up with maintenance every other month for a week at a time with the Verma-Plus and Para-Key products, just in case. Specific yeast-controlling products (Y-C Cleanse, for example) can also be utilized in this manner as can any of the supplements that help to ward off

Superbugs (like H. pylori, as discussed in Chapter 5). If you are using Dr. Ohhira's Probiotics 12 PLUS, you are way ahead of the game already.

Your diet plan this week will combine all the nutritional changes you made in weeks One and Two with a more liberal use of certain formerly off-limits foods, as well as introducing some extremely helpful healing substances that will help Feed the gut lining and help repair some of the damage the Colon Corruptors have inflicted. As in previous chapters, the Week Three shopping list for perishable foods immediately follows the meal plan. Let's review the six tactics that help Feed your gut and keep you radiantly healthy for life.

1. **Promote protein.** You'll eat at least eight ounces per day chosen from lean beef, poultry, and fish. To this you can add one to two of the omega-rich eggs for protein-packed snacks. Enjoy up to two whey-based protein drinks in addition to the basic protein requirement. Most individuals with lactose or casein allergies can tolerate the Fat Flush whey protein (see Resources), which is both lactose- and casein-free.

2. **Vitalize with veggies.** Enjoy at least five vibrant nonstarchy veggies per day, such as asparagus, zucchini, tomatoes, parsley, yellow squash, broccoli, cauliflower, red, green, and yellow peppers.

3. **Sweeten up with fruits.** You can now rotate back up to two fruits per day, which are perfect choices for smoothies or snacks. Choose from the low-sugar but satisfying apple (1), pear (1), berries (1 cup), plum (2), peach (1), nectarine (1), cherries (10), grapefruit (½), orange (1), avocado (½). (If diarrhea is still a challenge, please cook your fruits.) Also note that you can substitute half of a fruit exchange for one fruit juice–sweetened slice of bread or waffle for variety. See Chapter 10 for brand recommendations.

4. **Satisfy with starches.** Enjoy beans several times a week, favoring the garbanzos, adzuki, black beans, and lentils, which are high in minerals. Just remember that the harder beans must be presoaked for twenty-four hours to remove starchy residues that can create digestive discomfort.

5. **Add a Feeding beverage.** Beyond consuming half of your body weight in ounces of water during the day, drink two cups of tea made from healing/soothing slippery elm powder.

6. **Repair your gut with L-glutamine and deglycyrrhized licorice (DGL).**
   Help to heal any damage in the mucosal lining of the GI tract with
   L-glutamine (500–1,000 mg) at least twenty minutes before meals as well
   as approximately 380 mg deglycyrrhized licorice twenty minutes before
   meals, three times daily.

Sample Menu Plans for Week Three

DAY 1

BREAKFAST	*Strawberry Smoothie* 1 cup frozen strawberries blended with 1 serving whey protein powder, 8 ounces filtered water, 1 tablespoon lemon-flavored fish oil, ½ teaspoon vanilla extract, and a dash of ground cinnamon 1 *Almond Meal Muffin**
MIDMORNING SNACK	1 cup *Ann Louise's Yogurt** or plain whole-milk yogurt mixed with 1 tablespoon ground flaxseed and 1 tablespoon almond butter *(Use a teaspoon of Flora-Key for sweetener, if you like.)*
LUNCH	4 oz grilled or pan-fried turkey burger topped with ¼ cup broccoli sprouts and 1 tablespoon salsa 1 cup steamed asparagus sprinkled with 1 tablespoon toasted pine nuts and a pinch of dried oregano 2 cups *each* steamed red leaf and romaine lettuces, 5 olives, halved, 1 tablespoon chopped green onions, and 5 cherry tomatoes, tossed with 1 tablespoon *Lemon Caper Dressing** and 1 tablespoon *each* chopped basil and ground flaxseed
MIDAFTERNOON SNACK	2 hard-boiled eggs with 1 medium carrot ¼ cup chopped walnuts
DINNER	*Chicken Stir-fry* 4 oz chicken breast, cut into strips, stir-fried in 1 tablespoon sesame oil with 3 cups mixture chopped broccoli, onions, snow peas, red bell pepper, and zucchini, 1 tablespoon *each* minced garlic and ginger and a dash of salt served over ½ cup cooked brown rice pasta tossed with 2 teaspoons minced garlic and a dash of cayenne and sprinkled with toasted sesame seeds

Tip of the Day: *One cup fresh or frozen strawberries provides 94.12 mg vitamin C, 3.81 grams fiber, 44.82 IU vitamin A, and even 1 gram of protein. Welcome back, healthy fruit.*

DAY 2

BREAKFAST	½ grapefruit sprinkled with ground cinnamon
	½ cup cooked oatmeal mixed with 1 cup *Ann Louise's Yogurt** or plain whole-milk yogurt, 1 tablespoon *each* ground flaxseed and chopped walnuts, and a dash of ground ginger and cloves *(Use a teaspoon of Flora-Key for sweetener, if you like.)*
MIDMORNING SNACK	1 cup steamed cauliflower florets with 1 tablespoon *Ranch Dressing** and 2 tablespoons toasted pumpkin seeds
LUNCH	*Salmon Salad* 4 oz wild salmon (canned) tossed with 2 cups steamed chopped red cabbage, 2 teaspoons *each* minced red onion and chopped garlic, ¼ cup *each* chopped bell pepper, carrots, and celery, 1 tablespoon Vegenaise, and juice of 1 lime, topped with 2 tablespoons toasted sunflower seeds
	1 slice *Mega-Grain Quick Bread** sprinkled with ground cinnamon
MIDAFTERNOON SNACK	1 cup hot chicken broth with 1 teaspoon kelp powder
	1 pear
DINNER	*Turkey Marinara* 4 oz ground turkey sautéed in 1 tablespoon olive oil and tossed with 1 cup cooked spaghetti squash, 1 cup marinara sauce, 2 teaspoons *each* minced garlic and crushed fennel seed, 1 tablespoon *each* chopped fresh basil and oregano, a dash of salt and a pinch cayenne
	2 cups steamed green beans tossed with 1 tablespoon lemon-flavored fish oil and ½ teaspoon *each* dried dill and turmeric, topped with 1 chopped hard-boiled egg and 1 tablespoon toasted chopped almonds

Tip of the Day: Kelp powder is loaded with trace minerals like iodine and can be used not only as an addition to soups or broths but also as a seasoning or salt substitute.

DAY 3

BREAKFAST	2-egg omelet (cooked in 2 teaspoons of butter and a dash of salt) with 1 cup chopped fennel, 2 teaspoons minced garlic, and 1 tablespoon *each* chopped onion and toasted pine nuts, topped with 2 tablespoons salsa and ¼ teaspoon dried oregano 1 *Almond Meal Muffin**
MIDMORNING SNACK	*Raspberry-Almond Yogurt Smoothie* 1 cup frozen raspberries blended with 2 tablespoons almonds, 1 serving whey protein powder, 8 ounces filtered water, 1 cup *Ann Louise's Yogurt** or plain whole-milk yogurt, 1 tablespoon *each* ground flaxseed and flaxseed oil, and a pinch *each* ground cinnamon and cloves *(Use a teaspoon of* Flora-Key *for sweetener, if you like.)*
LUNCH	*Tuna Salad* 4 oz tuna (canned) in ½ avocado topped with 1 tablespoon *each* chopped green onion, carrots, and celery, and ½ cup mung bean sprouts, drizzled with 1 tablespoon lemon-flavored fish oil and sprinkled with 1 tablespoon chopped walnuts
MIDAFTERNOON SNACK	½ cup *each* red bell pepper and jicama sticks ½ cup *Garbanzo Bean Hummus** sprinkled with ¼ teaspoon ground cumin and a dash of cayenne
DINNER	1 cup *Creamy Kobocha Squash Soup** topped with 1 tablespoon ground flaxseed 4 oz pan-seared turkey tenderloins (seasoned with salt, garlic powder, and turmeric before cooking), topped with ¼ cup *Parsley Tahini Sauce** *(Prepare 8-oz turkey tenderloins so you have enough for tomorrow's lunch.)* 2 cups steamed kale with 1 tablespoon *each* minced shallot, garlic, and ginger, tossed with 1 tablespoon olive oil, 2 teaspoons apple cider vinegar, and splash of lemon

Tip of the Day: *Black beans, popular in Latin American recipes, are a great source of nutritional antioxidants, plant protein, fiber, and numerous other nutrients. If using dry beans, remember to soak them overnight in the refrigerator and rinse them several times to ensure release of hard-to-digest sugars.*

DAY 4

BREAKFAST	2 scrambled eggs (cooked in 2 teaspoons of butter and a dash of salt) 1 slice toasted rice pecan or other gluten-free bread (or *Mega-Grain Quick Bread**) spread with 1 tablespoon almond butter and sprinkled with 1 tablespoon ground flaxseed
MIDMORNING SNACK	2 stewed plums topped with 2 tablespoons ground walnuts and sprinkled with ground cinnamon and ginger
LUNCH	1 cup last night's *Creamy Kobocha Squash Soup** 4 oz last night's turkey tenderloins 1 cup steamed carrots and snow peas mixture ½ cup broccoli sprouts tossed with1 tablespoon lemon-flavored fish oil
MIDAFTERNOON SNACK	1 cup plain kefir mixed with a dash ground allspice and 1 tablespoon *each* ground almonds and ground flaxseed *(Use a teaspoon of Flora-Key for sweetener, if you like.)* 1 orange
DINNER	2 cups *Black Bean 'n' Beef Chili with a Twist** served over ½ cup cooked quinoa mixed with 2 teaspoons chopped garlic and a dash of salt (Make 1 cup cooked quinoa so you have enough for tomorrow's lunch.) *Simple Salad* 2 cups steamed romaine leaves, 4 artichoke hearts ½ cup *each* chopped cucumber and tomato, 2 tablespoons *each* chopped parsley and red onion, ½ teaspoon dried oregano, and a dash of cayenne tossed with 1 tablespoon *Lemon Caper Dressing**

Tip of the Day: *Cooking or stewing fruit will break down the cellulose, rendering the fruit more easily digested. Eating fruit while warm makes it more dessertlike, too!*

DAY 5

BREAKFAST	½ cup cooked oatmeal mixed with 1 cup *Ann Louise's Yogurt** or plain whole-milk yogurt, 1 tablespoon ground flaxseed, ½ apple, chopped, and 2 tablespoons sunflower seeds *(Use a teaspoon of Flora-Key for sweetener, if you like.)*
MIDMORNING SNACK	½ apple sliced sprinkled with ground cinnamon and ginger ¼ cup Brazil nuts
LUNCH	2 cups last night's *Black Bean 'n' Beef Chili with a Twist** served over ½ cup last night's cooked quinoa *Simple Salad* 4 slices avocado (half avocado total), 2 teaspoons chopped green onions, ¼ cup *each* chopped black olives and grated carrot, 1 cup broccoli sprouts, and 1 tablespoon pumpkin seeds drizzled with 1 tablespoon lemon-flavored fish oil
MIDAFTERNOON SNACK	2 hard-boiled eggs 1 slice toasted rice pecan or other gluten-free bread (or *Mega-Grain Quick Bread**) drizzled with 1 tablespoon coconut oil and sprinkled with ground cinnamon and 1 tablespoon ground almonds
DINNER	4 oz grilled wild salmon brushed with 1 tablespoon *Must Have Miso Dressing** 1 cup whole soybean pasta tossed with ½ cup *Parsley Tahini Sauce** 2 cups Swiss chard steamed with 2 teaspoons minced garlic and ¼ teaspoon turmeric, sprinkled with 1 tablespoon ground flaxseed and drizzled with 2 teaspoons apple cider vinegar

Tip of the Day: *Apple cider vinegar adds zippy flavor to your meals, is a great source of potassium, and has antibacterial and antifungal properties.*

DAY 6

BREAKFAST	*Veggie Scrambler* 2 eggs (cooked with 2 teaspoons of butter and a dash of salt) scrambled with ½ cup chopped broccoli, 2 tablespoons *each* chopped shallots and orange bell pepper, ¼ cup chopped tomato, and ½ teaspoon crushed fennel seeds, topped with 1 tablespoon chopped parsley and 1 tablespoon ground flaxseed
MIDMORNING SNACK	1 cup plain kefir mixed with a dash of ground cloves and cinnamon *(Use a teaspoon of Flora-Key for sweetener, if you like.)* 10 cherries (or 1 serving of another seasonal fruit) ¼ cup Brazil nuts
LUNCH	*Salmon Salad* 4 oz wild salmon (canned) mixed with 2 tablespoons *each* chopped celery, onion, and jicama and 1 tablespoon *Ranch Dressing** on bed of 2 cups steamed baby spinach *Vegetable Medley* 2 cups mixture steamed zucchini, carrots, and artichokes tossed with 1 teaspoon *each* minced ginger and garlic and 1 tablespoon *each* chopped cilantro and chives drizzled with 1 tablespoon lemon-flavored fish oil
MIDAFTERNOON SNACK	1 cup *Miso Soup Plus** topped with 1 tablespoon ground almonds and ¼ cup broccoli sprouts 2 tangerines
DINNER	4 oz grilled top sirloin (rubbed with garlic and sprinkled with salt, turmeric, and cayenne before cooking) 1 cup *each* grilled bell peppers and onions topped with ¼ teaspoon *each* dried oregano and thyme 1 small baked sweet potato topped with 1 tablespoon *each* coconut oil and ground flaxseed

Tip of the Day: Not only does coconut oil, with its medium-chain fats, aid in deactivating yeast and fungus, it is also an exceptional flavor-enhancing oil with weight-loss properties.

DAY 7

BREAKFAST	*Blueberry-Walnut Yogurt Smoothie* 1 cup frozen blueberries blended with 2 tablespoons walnuts, 1 serving whey protein powder, 8 oz filtered water, 1 cup *Ann Louise's Yogurt** or plain whole-milk yogurt, 1 tablespoon ground flaxseed, 1 tablespoon lemon-flavored fish oil, and a dash of ground cinnamon and cloves *(Use a teaspoon of Flora-Key for sweetener, if you like.)*
MIDMORNING SNACK	2 chopped hard-boiled eggs mixed with 1 tablespoon *Ranch Dressing** ½ cup sugar snap peas
LUNCH	*Sardine Salad* 4-oz can sardines packed in olive oil on a bed of 2 cups steamed baby spinach with ½ cup *each* chopped onion, cucumber, and jicama, 6 *each* halved black olives and cherry tomatoes, juice of ½ lime, and ¼ teaspoon dried oregano 1 *Almond Meal Muffin**
MIDAFTERNOON SNACK	½ cup *Garbanzo Bean Hummus** and ¼ cup broccoli sprouts rolled up in 4 large leaves of steamed lettuce
DINNER	*Baked Halibut in Parchment* 4 oz halibut fillet placed on parchment paper, topped with 1 tablespoon *Parsley and Cilantro Pesto** and 1 tablespoon *each* chopped orange bell pepper and tomato, sides of parchment paper folded in, ends tucked under, and baked at 375 degrees F. for 10–12 minutes, or until fish flakes ½ small baked delicata squash drizzled with 1 tablespoon coconut oil and sprinkled with a dash of curry powder, ground turmeric, and ginger 1 cup steamed asparagus tossed with juice of ½ lemon and 1 tablespoon *each* pumpkin seeds and ground flaxseed

Tip of the Day: Parchment paper is a must for the pantry. It is superior in gently steaming foods, holding in nutrition and flavor, as well as making a lovely presentation on your dinner plate.

Week Three Perishables Shopping List

This list includes all the perishables for Week Three of the Gut Flush Plan. (Note: The staples shopping list is located in Chapter 10, "Getting Ready for Gut Flush.")

Produce

Apple	1 medium
Cherries	¼ lb
Grapefruit	1
Lemons	About 5 (or as needed)
Limes	2 (or as needed)
Orange	1
Pear	1 small
Plums	2
Tangerines	2
Asparagus	1 lb
Avocado	1 medium
Bean sprouts	1 package
Beans, green	½ lb
Bell pepper, green	1
Bell pepper, orange	2
Bell pepper, red	2 to 3
Broccoli	1 head
Broccoli sprouts	1 package
Cabbage, green	1 medium head
Cabbage, red	1 medium head
Carrots, large	1 bunch or 1-lb bag
Cauliflower	1 small head
Celery	1 bunch
Cucumber	1 large
Garlic	2 heads (or as needed)
Ginger	1 small head (if needed)
Greens, fennel	1 small bunch

Greens, kale	1 small bunch
Greens, red leaf lettuce	1 small head
Greens, romaine	1 head
Greens, Swiss chard	1 bunch
Jerusalem artichoke	1 medium
Jicama	1 large
Mung bean sprouts	1 container
Onion, green	1 bunch
Onion, white or yellow	3 medium
Radish	1 bunch
Radish, daikon	1 small
Shallots	3
Snow peas	½ lb
Sugar snap peas	½ lb
Spinach, baby	3-oz bag
Squash, delicata	1 medium
Squash, kabocha	1 medium
Squash, spaghetti	1 medium
Squash, zucchini	2 medium
Sweet potato	1 small
Tomatoes	2 medium
Tomatoes, Cherry	½ pint
Yam	1 small
Basil	1 bunch
Chives	1 small bunch
Cilantro	1 bunch
Dill	1 small bunch
Mint	1 small bunch
Oregano	1 bunch
Parsley	1 bunch

Soy and Dairy

Miso, yellow	1 small container (if needed)
Tofu, soft (silken)	1 small container

Milk (whole or 2%)	2 quarts *(needed if making own yogurt)*
Yogurt, unsweetened, plain (whole or low-fat)	2 quarts *(needed if NOT making own yogurt)*

Lean Protein

Eggs	1 dozen
Beef, ground	1¼ lb
Beef, top sirloin	6 oz
Boneless, skinless chicken breast	2 5-oz breasts
Boneless, skinless turkey breast	8 oz
Ground turkey breast	6 oz (or 1 frozen 100% turkey burger)
Turkey tenderloins	10 oz
Halibut fillet	4 oz
Salmon fillet	4 oz

The Gut Flush
Plan for Life

14

Gut Flush at Home

You've completed the 21-Day Gut Flush Plan, and you're committed to lifelong health for your GI tract. You know that those Colon Corruptors are never going to stop looking for inroads into your life. While protecting your health and your gut with the best foods and supplements will take you a long way, you need to close the other gaps in your environment. That means having a Gut Healthy Home.

When you are creating a home environment that nurtures and encourages better health for your gut, your primary objective is to lessen your toxic load. When you decrease the toxic challenges to your system, your living quarters become your personal sanctuary where only health and healing rule. Home is the one place where you can truly be vigilant and proactive against Food Fright and the environmental dangers that surround us daily in the outside world. You have a great deal of control in preventing your house from becoming a toxic environment that breeds many of the health challenges I've been discussing throughout this book.

Simple measures, such as not allowing anyone to wear shoes in your home, can easily enhance your health and that of your family. Studies show that homes where people wear their shoes have higher levels of lead, pesticides, and other toxic contaminants, all tracked in by footwear. By merely having family members and visitors leave their shoes by the door, you significantly reduce environmental toxins in your home.

Your immune system is your body's best friend, but if it is busy fighting off heavy metals and pathogens in the air you breathe, it can easily become overloaded and drained. When this happens, those nasty yeast, parasites, and Superbugs can more easily become freeloading hitchhikers, something Gut Flushers are all determined to prevent.

In this chapter, you will discover myriad ways to reduce your home's impact on your total toxic load, from the kitchen to the bathroom, so you can further Fortify your defenses and achieve vital health. Please don't feel overwhelmed by the number of suggestions I offer here. Flushing your home is not meant to create mountains of extra work. And you certainly don't have to implement all of these measures at once. Just pick the easiest ones first, discuss them with your family members, and start there. The kitchen is a great place to begin.

Flushing the Kitchen

Your kitchen is a very important room in your house. In fact, it may be the *most* important one for putting into place proper safeguards to protect your digestive tract and implement the most critical aspects of the Gut Flush Plan.

As we have covered in chapters 6 and 7, the essential first step in the Gut Flush Plan is to remove all foods that contain sugar, artificial sweeteners, trans fats, yeast, mold, gluten (including all wheat-, rye-, and barley-based foods or foods that contain these grains), milk, and corn. Flush out the fridge, the freezer, and the pantry. Don't tempt yourself by keeping non–Gut Flush-friendly foods around, even if they are supposed to be there only for guests. No guest needs them, either. If you don't have these foods in the house, you won't be tempted to eat them.

Now on to sanitation, an often overlooked aspect of gut health. Follow these guidelines to make your kitchen part of your Gut Flush solution, not part of the problem.

Wash your hands. As soon as you enter the kitchen, make it your habit to head directly to the sink. Never handle food with unwashed hands. The

Centers for Disease Control and Prevention has called hand washing "the single most important means of preventing the spread of infection."

Use probiotic soap. I have become a great fan of Dr. Ohhira's Kampuku soap, which is made with probiotics (see Resources). This soap provides you with the same antibacterial power on the outside of your body as the probiotics do internally. You should wash your hands thoroughly for twenty seconds. Some experts recommend washing for at least as long as it takes to sing "Happy Birthday" twice.

Use filtered water in the whole house. And this is especially important in the kitchen. Use a home water filter that cleans out organisms .05 microns and larger. Make sure the filter is certified to block parasitic cysts. As I've discussed previously, a Doulton water filter is my personal choice (see Resources).

Ventilate to the outdoors. Make sure the stove and oven are well vented to eliminate pollutants from cooking.

Maintain clean surfaces. Regularly disinfect surfaces that people frequently touch. These include door handles, phones, remote controls, and computer keyboards. Use a disinfectant like Lysol disinfectant spray. Otherwise, research shows, viruses and bacteria can survive on these surfaces in significant amounts for up to eighteen hours. Better still, consider using the Germ Control 24 product sold through Home Depot that is designed to kill MRSAs. I use this product as the final act in my housecleaning routine.

Prevent dishwashing mold. After cleaning dishes, dry them with a clean washcloth or let them air-dry in the dish rack. Don't stack dishes wet, as that can foster the growth of bacteria on the dishes.

Use separate cutting boards for meats and vegetarian foods. After handling raw meat, wash your hands and clean all surfaces touched by the meat with soap and water or a solution of one teaspoon of Clorox per quart of water. Rinse thoroughly. (Raw meat may contain a long list of dangerous pathogens, including H. pylori, E. coli, Salmonella, and Shigella, not to mention worms.)

Don't use unlined copper or any aluminum pots or pans. Copper destroys vitamin C and is antagonistic to zinc, one of your best mineral protectors against parasites. Aluminum can affect digestion by destroying the precious protein-digestive enzyme pepsin in the stomach. Instead of aluminum foil for cooking and reheating, use parchment paper. Invest in cookware that cooks by the minimum moisture method at 180 degrees—the temperature that kills germs and parasites but not vitamins and minerals. Check out Salad Master, available through saladmaster.com.

Throw out all cracked dishes. Bacteria can live in the cracks of cups and plates. These bacteria will mix with hot beverages or foods, creating digestive problems.

Replace or bleach wooden cutting and chopping boards. Again, bacteria can live in the cracks of wooden blocks. Use a Lucite chopping board or give your wooden boards a Clorox rinse (use approximately one teaspoon of Clorox to a quart of water and rinse well). You can also clean other utensils with the same solution.

Change and wash your dishcloths daily. Wet cloths are welcoming homes to bacteria and mold. And above all, please don't use sponges—the holes harbor bacteria and mold that you can't get out, even if you boil them.

Wash your forks with extra care. Research has shown that cheese fragments and other dairy products stuck to forks can be home to significant bacteria growth.

Don't forget the Gut Flush Food Bath. Remember to soak all foods including vegetables, fruits, chicken, fish, meats, and eggs with the special Gut Flush Food Bath (see page 37 for instructions). (*Note:* When you "bathe" your food, salads and raw veggies are fine at home, but I would not recommend them in restaurants where you don't know who has been handling—or mishandling—your foods.)

Lower the thermostat in your fridge and freezer. Set your refrigerator at 40 degrees Fahrenheit or lower and set your freezer at zero degrees or lower.

Don't sample foods before they're finished cooking. The fear of Salmonella got you over your raw cookie dough habit years ago, right? The same rationale extends to other foods. Enough said.

Cook all protein foods thoroughly. Always set the oven to at least 325 degrees Fahrenheit. When using a conventional oven, use a meat thermometer to make sure meats reach an adequately high internal temperature. Cook ground meat until no pink color is left, and hamburger meat and casseroles should reach 160 degrees Fahrenheit in the center. The internal temperature of roasts and steaks should reach at least 165 degrees; pork, 170 degrees; and poultry, 180 degrees. Cook eggs until both yolks and whites are firm. Cook fish in a conventional oven until it's flaky and white; bake at 400 degrees Fahrenheit for at least eight minutes per inch of thickness

And please don't ever cook beef, pork, or fish in a microwave. You can use it for reheating but not initial cooking.

Be cautious with leftovers. If you don't eat hot foods right away, keep them at 140 degrees or higher, or refrigerate immediately for later consumption. Reheat leftovers to at least 165 degrees Fahrenheit. Raw meat and poultry should be cooked within two days of purchase, or they should be frozen.

Banish pests. I think this goes without saying, but I've been to enough summertime parties where I see people ignoring this basic guideline: keep flies and other insects off food. They can transfer parasites when they land on foodstuffs.

Also, roach droppings lead to allergies. Use nontoxic roach traps to eliminate these bothersome pests, but don't use pesticides in the house.

Be liberal with that salt shaker. Stash a salt shaker and/or grinder next to the stove for regular use. As we talked about in Week One, salt has an antiseptic effect on bodily tissues.

And last but not least:

Never eat homemade sushi. Fine sushi restaurants employ well-trained chefs who have learned how to "candle" fish and extract undesirable larvae and the like. Chances are you don't have the training. Please leave sushi to the experts—or leave it alone altogether.

Flushing the Indoor Air

Next to flushing out the kitchen, the second most important step you need to take to reduce your overall toxic load is to protect your immediate environment against allergens, dust, and dust mites in the air you breathe. In many homes and buildings, the indoor air contains more problematic substances and organisms than outdoor air.

Use dehumidifiers. Dehumidifiers lower indoor humidity of damp air that would otherwise encourage the growth of mold, mildew, and bacteria. Use a dehumidifier during the humid winter months or in basements or other areas that tend to become damp.

Select a quality air filter. Air filters are most important in the most-frequented rooms in the house, the kitchen and the bedroom. In my home, I use the Bio-Net air purifier. Laboratory tested, this device has been listed by the FDA as a Class II Medical Device. The company claims that as air passes through the product's patented EGF germ-killing zone the first time, more than 99 percent of viruses and 94 to 100 percent of other microorganisms are reduced. In contrast, air filters that use HEPA and ultraviolet (UV) are not as effective. For example, HEPA-only air filters that claim 0.1 to 0.3 micron particle capture cannot kill and may not trap all viruses. Additionally, UV is not always strong enough to inactivate many other germs, and/or the germs may become shielded behind dirt particles and may not be killed.

Wash all clothing in hot water. Use water that is at least 140 degrees Fahrenheit. Researchers have found that washing at that temperature is the only way to kill all dust mites and effectively eliminate pet dander and pollen. So-called anti-mite additives are no better than using hot water with normal detergent.

Maintain bare floors. Get rid of carpets, especially wall-to-wall carpets. If you do want to have rugs, use throw rugs that you can launder. Carpeting attracts dust mites and allergens. Studies on rugs show that vacuuming them can't eliminate all contaminants. If you do vacuum rugs, use vacuum cleaners with rotating heads and HEPA filters for more effective cleaning.

Repair leaks. Leaky roofs and walls lead to accumulated dampness that allows the growth of fungus and mold. Aside from needlessly wasting water, leaky faucets add to the humidity of your house.

Strategically leave on lights. If you have mold or mildew growing in a closet or other dark area, leave a light on—light kills and inhibits fungi. Select low-wattage or environmentally sound fluorescent bulbs to save on energy.

Cut down foliage like ivy that grows on outside walls. They attract rodents which may enter the house, increasing the risk of increase allergies and asthma. Plant life near and around the outside of the house can also damage the walls and foundation of your home, creating leaks that admit moisture.

But add indoor plants. Houseplants like spider plants in the house can help clean indoor air.

Select furniture and window coverings carefully. Dispose of upholstered furniture and replace with leather or vinyl items. Use window shades, not venetian blinds, which are dust collectors. Also, wash or dust the shades regularly. Studies show that Superbugs can live on polyester drapes for up to seven weeks.

Dust and air out often. Dust furniture at least once a week with a damp cloth. Ventilate the house when you dust. In fact, open windows to let fresh air in as often as possible. Don't keep your home sealed up tight. Of course, if asthma or allergies are a major concern, you may wish to simply use air-conditioning and air filters instead of opening the windows.

Don't allow smoking in or near the house. Tobacco smoke is a well-documented source of toxins that cause heart disease, cancer, and diabetes. Of course you will not allow smoking within the house, but if guests want to smoke, send them across the street. Even smoking just *near* the house allows smoke to infiltrate the indoor air. Take all measures to avoid allowing family members to be exposed to secondhand smoke anywhere.

Clean the air cleaners. If you have filters in your heating/cooling system, change or clean them at least once a month. Dirty or clogged filters reduce air flow and efficiency, and they can even cause the system to break down entirely.

Have your house checked for radon. This radioactive gas is linked to lung cancer and is present in many houses. (It comes in from basements.) If your radon level is high, seal up cracks in your house's foundation where the gas may be coming in.

Keep the outdoors outdoors. Keeping the grass cut short around your house and in all outdoor areas where people and pets congregate will lower the risk of insect bites and ticks. After time spent outdoors check all family members for ticks and allergic reactions (like poison ivy rashes). Eliminate plants growing near the house to which family members are sensitive.

Finish those lingering home improvement projects. Your first priority is to eliminate old, chipping paint that may contain lead and give off lead-contaminated dust.

Flushing the Bedroom

Your bedroom may present special problems for health. Think of it: What do you do during sleep other than inhale the contents of air in your bedroom, over and over? Since you and your family spend over one-third of your life in the bedroom, contaminants in these rooms have a greater chance of being inhaled, raising your exposure to pollutants and thereby increasing the toxic load on your body. To gain the optimal benefit of sleep's restorative power, you must make your bedroom a sanctuary of health.

Don't forget that air filter! As I mentioned previously, the top priority in Flushing your bedroom should be to purchase a high-quality air filter, such as the Bio-Net air purifier (see description in "Select a quality air filter," on page 192). With so many options on the market, it may be tempting to buy a cheaper product, but I ask you to please value your health enough to pay the extra money for a brand of air filter that really works.

Use hypoallergenic bed linens. Don't sleep with nonwashable covers like sheepskins. Instead, choose a high-quality grade of cotton. Use dust mite–resistant covers on your pillows and hypoallergenic casings over your mattresses.

Protect your "sleep hygiene." Sleep should be a time of complete rest and absolutely no stress. Make the most of the curative power of sleep by aiming for seven to eight hours of total sleep every night. Try to go to bed and wake up at the exact same time every day. (The weekend sleep-in may seem like a good idea, but it can throw your body's natural rhythms out of sync.) Don't go to bed hungry, but don't eat a heavy meal within two hours of bedtime either. Eliminate all caffeine. Keep your bedroom dark, quiet, and slightly cool—a cracked window is an excellent way to get your daily quota of fresh air into your lungs, all year round.

Don't sleep right next to your clock radio. While no one has definitively proven that the electromagnetic field given off by this device causes harm, it does emit low levels of electromagnetic radiation. Why take a chance? Place it across the room or replace it with a battery-operated analog clock.

Flushing the Bathroom

The humidity in most bathrooms is ideal for the growth of fungi and bacteria, and the most common cleaning solutions used in bathrooms can be hazardous. Your best offense is a good, preventative defense. Try these tips to avoid some of the biggest risk factors.

Keep the air as clean and dry as possible. Frequently open bathroom windows to change the air and reduce humidity. Ventilate the bathroom very well when cleaning—keep the air moving by using a strong fan and opening the windows. Researchers have found that when you clean with only moderate ventilation—for instance, when removing accumulated residue off the shower wall—you can inhale three times the emissions limit set by the California Office of Environmental Health Hazard Assessment.

Designate his/her towels. To avoid the unfortunate sharing of bacteria, every member of the family should have an individual towel. Researchers have found that Superbugs and pubic lice (ew!) can be passed on by contact with towels.

Clean faucet handles often. In studies of bacteria on surfaces in houses and offices, faucet handles were near the top in levels of bacterial contamination.

Throw away that antibacterial soap. As we discussed previously, antibacterial soap merely encourages the development of antibiotic-resistant bacteria. Besides, research cited in the *Annals of Internal Medicine* shows that they don't protect from infections any more than plain old, normal soap. As a natural alternative, consider using Dr. Ohhira's probiotics Kampuku soap, which features herbs and plant extracts such as mulberry, Chinese cabbage, and wild strawberry that were combined and allowed to naturally ferment to create probiotics.

Don't use air fresheners. When the chemicals in air fresheners interact with ozone, they create airborne formaldehyde. And ozone can be pretty hard to avoid. (This tip is particularly important in your office bathroom, as ozone is also found in computer printers, fax machines, and copiers.)

Make sure the men in your life wash their hands. While 90 percent of women wash their hands after using the bathroom, only 75 percent of men do.

Microwave your dentures. If you use dentures that do not contain metal, put them in the microwave for two minutes at night to kill pathogens. Otherwise, contaminated dentures can lead to fungal infections of the mouth. Follow these guidelines for microwaving dentures:

1. Put dentures (that contain no metal) in microwave container with a vented cover that's at least twice as tall as the dentures.
2. Fill container with water.

3. Put tablet of denture cleanser in water.
4. Drape towel over microwave container's cover to absorb water.
5. Run microwave for two minutes.
6. Let dentures cool, then rinse.

Brush and floss teeth daily to remove food. These basics of oral hygiene minimize plaque and bacterial growth in the mouth. If not removed daily, plaque irritates gums and can lead to periodontal disease, which makes you more vulnerable to heart disease and infections. When brushing, brush in a circular motion (brushing horizontally exerts extra wear and tear on tooth enamel).

Flushing Your Pets

I am not arguing that pets can be a great health benefit. Research shows that pet owners have lower blood pressure and reduced stress when compared with people without pets. But pets can also be sources of parasites and other Colon Corruptors and can pass these pests on to humans. Enjoy your dogs, cats, and other animals, but use these guidelines to ensure the strict hygiene that is necessary in the handling of pets.

Keep pets out of your bedroom. Though you may not like to exclude them, pet hair and dander have no place in your bed. Plus, their restless nocturnal wanderings can disturb your sleep—and you need your rest more than they do. They sleep all day!

Bathe your pets (and your hands) regularly. If your pets go outdoors, consider a weekly bath to bar entry of any hitchhikers from the outdoors. And always wash your hands and your children's hands after they touch pets. Do *not* allow your dog to give "kisses"—contrary to that old wives' tale, dogs' mouths are teeming with bacteria.

Control your pet's pests. Deworm pets regularly. If you're concerned about toxic medicines, you can use half the dosage of both Verma-Plus and Para-Key. And even though you may be concerned about fleas, don't let pets wear flea collars. Pesticide residues in the pets' fur can be spread to members of the family.

Make kitty litter Dad's job. Don't let women of childbearing age clean kitty litter. It can be infected with toxoplasmosis, which is linked to birth defects. This parasite is also a danger to people with compromised immunity. Once a month, take indoor kitty litter boxes outside and clean them out thoroughly.

Flushing the Laundry

Researchers who have investigated how we do our laundry have discovered that washing machines and laundry rooms can be breeding grounds for bacteria, parasites, and other health dangers. Our habit of washing clothes in cold or lukewarm water has added to this problem. Here are some ways to flush pathogens from your laundry.

Wash bed linens effectively. To get rid of undesirable critters on a regular basis, wash all bedding, including comforters, in hot water (140 degrees Fahrenheit or hotter) at least once a week. Wash pillows every two weeks. If you're a parent, be sure to wash the stuffed toys that your children sleep with at least once a week.

Wash underwear separately. Underwear is often contaminated with microscopic bits of fecal matter, which you don't want spreading to other clothing or bedroom sheets. To minimize possible contamination, launder underwear as the last load of wash, and always use water that's at least 140 degrees Fahrenheit.

Again, wash your hands! Always wash your hands after handling laundry. A study from the American Society for Microbiology found that wet clothes from the washing machine often contain bacteria and viruses.

Clean the machines. To disinfect your washing machine, once a week, run a cycle with just Clorox in the machine, no clothing. Make sure your dryer is well vented to keep dust and lint from entering indoor air.

Know when to ditch your clothes. Be especially careful in handling clothes that may be contaminated with the sap from poison ivy, poison oak, or poison sumac. You can suffer an allergic reaction to these substances. Hats, jackets, and gloves that may have been exposed to these plants need to be laundered before being worn again.

Flushing the Metals

Today more than ever, our bodies are bombarded by pesticides, chemicals, and other environmental pollutants that leave us increasingly vulnerable to a host of disorders that will only compound your Gut Flush challenges. Heavy metals are another hidden threat to health. While I have covered some of them briefly above, here's more info on specific minerals—where you'll find them and how to Flush them from your life.

Flush aluminum. Don't take antacids which, aside from inhibiting valuable stomach acid (HCl) that protects you against a variety of pathogens, may contain excess aluminum. Other sources of aluminum include antiperspirants and cosmetics, as well as aluminum pots and pans. Early signs that you may have been overexposed to aluminum include dry skin, heartburn, flatulence, vulnerability to catching colds, colic, memory loss, Parkinson's symptoms, muscle weakness, and mental confusion. Using an infrared sauna can help your body sweat out heavy metals.

Flush arsenic. Arsenic can be a common contaminant in drinking water. Have your water tested, especially if you use a well. But you may also be exposed to arsenic in smoke from a stove that burns wood treated with arsenic-laced additives. If you heat with a wood-burning stove, make sure the room is well ventilated. In addition, keep these sources of arsenic out of your indoor air: tobacco smoke, coal dust, insecticides, herbicides, and paints. Inhaling arsenic can cause severe coughing, breathing difficulties, restlessness, and cyanosis—a bluish pallor to the skin.

You can check your fingernails for signs of arsenic poisoning—it leaves horizontal white bands or longitudinal brown bands on fingernails and toenails. It can also discolor nails, making them brownish, or cause nail loss. Other signs of long-term arsenic ingestion include skin discolorations, diarrhea, vomiting, nausea, peripheral nerve damage, deafness, memory loss, confusion, uncoordinated movement, and visual problems.

Flush copper. Copper overload can compromise your adrenal function and your nervous system. Experts like Dr. Paul C. Eck of the Analytical Research Laboratories in Phoenix suspect that we ingest too much copper from birth control pills, dental fillings, copper intrauterine devices, and the fungicides applied to food and added to the water in swimming pools. In addition, copper-rich foods include nuts, seeds, avocados, grains, shellfish, chocolate, tea, wheat germ bran, and brewer's yeast.

Possible symptoms of copper toxicity can include insomnia, anorexia, obsessive-compulsive behavior, skin abnormalities, hyperactivity, loss of hair, allergies, and depression. If you suspect you suffer from too much copper, consider a tissue mineral analysis (TMA; see Resources).

Flush lead. Lead contamination has been a problem for people ever since wine in ancient Rome leached lead from pottery. The Environmental Protection Agency estimates that nearly half a million children have too much lead in their bodies. Lead is especially damaging to the brain and nervous system. It retards mental development, reduces intelligence, and can lead to attention deficit disorder and hyperactivity.

Sources of lead in the house include chips of decaying paint, water that picks up lead from lead pipes, some toys, food packaging, and electrical cords. Be alert to news reports of recalls of children's toys that contain too much lead.

Symptoms of lead poisoning include behavioral problems, blue gums, loss of hearing, visual disturbances, stomach pain, menstrual irregularities, miscarriages, kidney disease, and convulsions. In extreme cases, lead poisoning is fatal.

Flush mercury. Mercury is used in dental fillings, batteries, and thermometers (though the introduction of electric thermometers has reduced this usage). Symptoms of mercury exposure include kidney malfunction, dementia, heart disease, compromised immunity, mood swings, memory loss, fatigue, and headaches.

To limit your mercury exposure, have your silver fillings removed by a dentist experienced at the safe removal of dental amalgams, don't eat larger fish like tuna or swordfish, and avoid freshwater fish.

Flushing Your Life

As you may have guessed, cleanliness is your best protection against the Superbugs and other pathogens that are so threatening to health. I don't mean that you should become totally neurotic about germs. Germs are omnipresent. You can't escape them and you shouldn't try to live in a totally sterile environment because you never will. But basic measures must be taken to ensure that your home environment is protected and that sources of contamination are Flushed out of your life. I know you'll find, like so many of my clients, that the benefits outweigh the bother of changing your home to protect yourself and your loved ones.

What's harder to control is the big wide world beyond our front door. Let's take a look at how you can control as many of the toxic-loading variables as possible while you are on the road.

15

Gut Flush on the Road

Please don't let the reality of today's world being full of Food Frights and Superbugs take the wind out of your sails. Actually, with a little enlightened planning and practical understanding of what the dangers are out there in unfamiliar territory, you can still have a wonderful time, remain healthy, and return home safe and sound. You just have to be prepared—more so today than ever before—to protect and defend yourself against the Colon Corruptors.

In addition to your primary objective while at home—to lower the toxic load on your body—you must also simultaneously mount a serious defense against incoming invaders. The biggest threats while traveling come from your food and water, but pathogens can also sneak in during some otherwise innocuous moments, whether it is flushing the toilet or signing your credit card slip in the checkout line as you will learn about in a moment. Let's take a look at some of the most prevalent—and the sneakiest—hidden risks and how you can protect your gut in your travels.

Dining on the Road

When you travel, you have to choose your food wisely, very wisely. While the ideal situation would be for you to bring your specially bathed food from home, this is usually impractical. Besides, going out to eat is part of the fun in traveling. Instead of holing up in your hotel room with a box of gluten-free crackers, try a few of these strategies to stay safe.

Eat only well-cooked foods. Period. Regardless of all other precautions, your first basic precaution in order to dodge a food-borne illness is to never, I repeat *never,* eat raw foods or undercooked foods when traveling abroad or in areas where the food is likely to be infected. No matter how reliable the source seems to be, raw food presents the highest risk of making you sick.

Anything raw or undercooked, like meat, shellfish, or fish, is often seething with pathogens and parasites that can infect your digestive tract. Plus, undercooked food or cooked food that has been at room temperature for a few hours may also present other dangers.

You should only eat food that has been cooked while you wait and that is still piping hot. *Remember that bacteria start to multiply like crazy after two hours. (Make that every hour in the summertime.) Even after the two-hour period, many strains of bacteria multiply every twenty minutes thereafter, even on cooked food.*

Skip the salad. Including fruit salad. Especially when you're traveling in a relatively undeveloped country, don't eat vegetables that are not extremely well cooked. Don't touch raw salads, no matter how well washed. Personally, I wouldn't eat fruit, even if you peel it first, unless that fruit is a banana. (I have analyzed way too many diet diaries of individuals who have picked up an "uninvited guest" during their travels. The common denominator in all these diet histories was "peeled" fresh fruit.)

And, by all means, skip the salad bar. Serve-yourself salad and food bars, in any country, are just colorful buffets of bacteria. First of all, the food literally sits out for hours. Dishes are often "married" together, meaning that restaurant workers combine leftover, already spoiling food with fresh hot food in a continual round robin of bacteria. Perhaps most troubling, countless people reach in and touch the food that you'll eventually bring to your lips. Years ago at a brunch buffet, I saw a man grab a sticky bun, lick every single one of his fingers, and then reach underneath the "sneeze guard" for another, touching several other baked goods, before ultimately deciding against seconds. Please, trust me on this.

Ditch dairy. Since you're avoiding milk on the Gut Flush Plan already, please try to stay away from dairy on the road as well. In particular, don't consume unpasteurized milk or dairy products like cheese, as these can frequently be contaminated with Shigella.

Do a covert kitchen inspection. You should also be mindful of cooked food that has been contaminated by unsanitary handling techniques. If you can, take a peek into the kitchen and watch the way food is being prepared. If you've decided to brave a salad, check to make sure that gloves are worn by the salad makers.

Dust your food. I often take along some powdered charcoal from activated charcoal capsules, my very own stash of "chardust," which can be sprinkled on foods you suspect could be less than pure.

Don't eat off the street. Along with this advice, remember to avoid consuming drinks or food bought from street vendors. They are often contaminated with pathogens.

Choose specific ethnic foods. The safest restaurants to frequent would be Italian, Greek, Moroccan, Turkish, Lebanese, and Indian because of the rich use of pathogen-fighting garlic, oregano, and cayenne used in these cuisines.

Be wary of seafood. The CDC warns that many people have become sick from eating seafood brought back from overseas. In particular, the CDC reports that people have come down with cholera from crab carried back from Latin America. Approach seafood with caution, and consider avoiding it altogether until you are back home.

Use hand gel before every meal. To help ensure that you don't accidentally contaminate your own food, travel with a cleansing hand gel that contains more than 60 percent alcohol. Always use it to clean your hands before eating. In addition, clean with the gel after going to the bathroom, touching animals or pets, changing diapers, or coming into contact with young children.

Protect your baby's food source. Infants less than six months old who travel should be breast-fed for the safest source of food. But if a child has already stopped breast-feeding, cook up formula from a commercial powder with boiled water.

Eat before a plane flight. I've always known that having a little something to eat or drink before a flight (it's nearly impossible to eat healthfully on planes these days, as we all know) made me feel better because it raised blood sugar levels, which also balanced my mood. But now researchers have found that a snack before takeoff is healthy for a different reason. Eating raises your blood volume and can keep you from feeling light-headed or having circulatory problems when you're airborne. Food and drink protects you against the negative effects of the low pressure in the airplane cabin at high altitudes. Try pumpkin seeds, which will not only parasite-proof your body but also provide fats, protein, and carbs for blood sugar regulation. (If the truth be told, I have even been known to chew on Dr. Ohhira's Probiotics 12 PLUS for food. After all, it is fermented from ninety-two plants, herbs, and fruits.)

But not **on** *the plane.* The CDC cautions that you shouldn't assume that water and food on a commercial airliner is always safe to consume. Those items may have originated in the country from which a flight takes off. So you should assume they could be contaminated and not eat or drink them.

Drinking on the Road

Between the food you eat and the water you drink, you could run into some really unpleasant bacteria and parasites out there. Those most commonly contracted by travelers include Shigella (bacillary dysentery), E. coli, cryptosporidium, hepatitis A, amoeba, Giardia, and norovirses. But you can also pick up Salmonella, typhoid fever, rotavirus infections, and cholera, as well as a host of other nasty protozoan parasites, depending on where you travel.

Access to clean water takes you a far way toward mitigating your risks. Try to follow as many of these tips as possible—if not all of them.

Go for recognizable brands. As a general rule, when you're traveling in places where the water is iffy, only drink liquids you can really be sure of: bottled water of a brand you recognize (make sure it hasn't been opened), wine, beer, tea, or coffee prepared with boiled water, or soft drinks and carbonated mineral water that hasn't previously been opened.

Skip the glass or cup. In all cases, it's better to drink beverages right out of the bottle or can rather than a container whose cleanliness you're not sure of. You also have to watch out for water sitting on the outside of cans and bottles—even that may have pathogens. So use a sanitizing wipe to clean the outside of the container, and make sure everything is clean and dry before you put your mouth on a bottle or can.

No juice or smoothies. Stay away from fruit juice that has been made with local water and fruit. If a local water supply is treated with chlorine that meets the kind of standards used in the United States, it should be free of viruses and bacteria. Still, chlorine doesn't kill parasites like cryptosporidium, amoeba, or Giardia.

Drink it without ice. Ice in beverages may also be contaminated. Plus, if there's been ice in your glass, bottle, cup, or other container you are going to drink out of, get rid of the ice and clean that container with hot water and soap.

Boil water for absolute safety. Boiling your water is considered the best way to kill most of the commonly encountered pathogens and make water safer for drinking. Bring it to a strong boil for at least five minutes and then let it cool down to room temperature. But don't add ice to cool it off. That just defeats the purpose of boiling. To make it taste a little better and relieve the flatness of boiled water, you can add a pinch of salt or pour it back and forth between clean containers (that aerates the water).

Always boil and filter water from lakes, reservoirs, ponds, rivers, and other outdoor sources before drinking. If you camp out, bring a portable water filter designed to filter out Giardia.

Use bottled water to brush your teeth. Don't brush your teeth with water that might be contaminated. Even the small amount that you use to rinse your toothbrush could be enough to infect you.

Use iodine sparingly. The CDC recommends using iodine to disinfect questionable water, although iodine doesn't eliminate cryptosporidium. Plus, if your water is cloudy, it needs to be strained through a clean cloth (into a clean container) to get out whatever is floating in your water. Generally speaking, only after it is strained should it be treated with iodine.

The two best types of iodine to use are an iodine tincture and tetraglycine hydroperiodide tablets, which can be bought at sporting-good stores and drugstores. When you use these products, follow the package instructions to the letter. If you do have to treat cloudy water, you have to use twice as many tablets. If the water is very cold (less than about 42 degrees Fahrenheit), it should be warmed up to allow the iodine to work more effectively. Also iodine needs more time to disinfect water if the water is cloudy.

If you do travel in a place where you have to use iodine to treat your water, use it for only a few weeks. More than that and you risk taking in too much iodine, which can play havoc with your thyroid.

Get a good portable filter, use it carefully, and don't share. Generally, the portable filters you can use to filter water are designed to be used along with a disinfection chemical like iodine to eliminate most pathogens. While reverse-osmosis filters are effective at taking out bacteria, protozoan parasites, and viruses, they cost a lot and are cumbersome. Their other main disadvantage: the small holes in these porous systems are quickly clogged by water that contains a lot of sediment. Chlorine may also ruin their membranes.

Since filters are designed to take pathogens out of water, be cautious when changing filters. Wash your hands when you are done.

For the best safety, don't entrust your filter to anyone else. If a filter is put in wrong or isn't changed often enough, it could fail to remove pathogens. In addition, you should inspect the filter cartridges. Poor quality in the manufacturing process may allow some parasites or other organisms to get through. Don't use a filter cartridge that looks bad. Replace the cartridges according to the manufacturer's recommended calendar.

Lowering Your Toxic Load When Traveling

Beyond food and water, there are thousands of other ways Colon Corruptors can hop aboard and end up ruining a fun trip. You're not a party pooper if you take precautions—you're a smart traveler. Check out some of these ways to safeguard your long-term health by avoiding pathogens away from home.

About Town

Your trip needn't take you around the globe to put you in harm's way. You may be surprised to learn that sometimes, the most "gut-threatening" locations are right around the corner.

Use antiseptic spray on equipment at the gym. Studies of gym equipment have found evidence of Superbugs growing on dumbbells and benches. Many gyms have squeeze bottles of spray cleaners and paper towels available—use them. Wipe down any surface you may touch, even briefly.

Keep your nails short and trim them often. Superbugs have been found to hide under longer fingernails—don't give them another place to take up residence.

Use your own pen. When you're at the bank or in the checkout line, you may be tempted to use the pen attached to the cord to sign your checks or credit card receipt. Don't—it may be teeming with bacteria. Make a habit of using your own pen in all such public signing areas.

Step away from a flushing toilet. The spray from a toilet flush can splatter residue of Superbugs like E. coli. Get away from the toilet as quickly as possible once you press the handle to flush.

Wash children's hands when leaving a petting zoo. Otherwise, they can pick up parasites and infections. Recently petting zoos experienced outbreaks of E. coli, Salmonella, and cryptosporidium. Also, if you have a baby or toddler, keep pacifiers tucked away in a sealed plastic bag while in the park and keep close watch to prevent any fingers from finding their way into mouths before you can find your way to a sink.

Disinfect your hotel room. Remember those scary reports of what *really* lurks on the hotel bedspreads? Well, every surface of a hotel room is the same—phone receivers, TV remotes, temperature dials, door handles, the bathroom counters, you name it. Make it a habit to walk through and wipe down every surface you might touch with antiseptic wipes, and keep wiping. And *never* use the glasses on the sink—recent undercover reports found that even at upscale hotels those glasses are rarely even cleaned, let alone sanitized, between guests.

Don't share your phone. A microbiologist at the University of Arizona in Tucson found that 50 percent of the cell phones he examined tested positive for MRSA. Don't lend yours out, and don't borrow anyone else's.

Apply hand gel, early and often. A few small travel-size bottles of alcohol-based hand gel, stashed in your coat pocket, purse, or gym bag, will keep them handy for you throughout the day. Whether it's using a handrail to board a bus, sliding your hand on a banister, punching sticky buttons in an elevator, exchanging money at the newsstand—you name it, you have countless reasons to apply the hand gel daily. Get the moisturizing kind so you don't dry out your hands with repeated applications.

At the Water's Edge

Swimming and bathing are particularly hazardous recreational activities for the unwary traveler. A slew of infections can be picked up by swimming in freshwater lakes, rivers and streams, saltwater oceans, bays, inlets, and tributaries and even swimming pools. As a matter of fact, just wading can lead to infections of the eyes, ears, nose, throat, skin, and lungs as well as diarrhea-causing GI infections and even nerve infections. At the same time, you are at increased risk if you put your head under water.

The problem begins with the pollutants that frequently get into water: sewage, agricultural runoff, animal waste products, and even dead animals. When feces get flushed into water, pathogens that convey waterborne disease can make you sick and give you severe diarrhea. A big part of the problem is the fact that it's just impossible to swim without swallowing a bit of water. (Be kind—please don't go swimming where you can spread your illness to fellow bathers.)

The most dangerous swimming situations and times are:

- a beach that is near farms or areas that contain livestock or domestic pets;
- swimming areas near storm drains that empty into the water;
- right after a heavy rainfall; that increases polluted runoff into water;
- freshwater bodies of water in Asia, Africa, the Caribbean, and South America that are known to have schistosomiasis (parasite infection caused by trematode worms);

- water where animals infected with Leptospira (bacterial disease that attacks the kidneys) frequently urinate;
- when you have a cut or wound that makes you more vulnerable to disease organisms getting into your body;
- near an industrial plant that empties warmed or heated water.

Even swimming pools filled with plenty of chlorine may still be home to Giardia and cryptosporidium. But if you feel like you must swim in a hotel pool, you can bring along testing kits with strips that check the chlorine levels in pools as well as their acidity to see if they are adequate to make it safe from most pathogens.

Buzzing in the Air

If you travel to an area that has malaria or other parasites/diseases passed by insects, insect repellant should be a priority in your campaign against Colon Corruptors. To avoid all manner of insectborne pathogens, follow these guidelines:

Go for the big gun: DEET. I don't know of anything "natural" that really works. What I do know, however, is that the CDC recommends DEET. The relatively minor risk of using the chemical DEET is nothing compared to the risk of mosquito stings.

Use enough for complete coverage but not overkill. Spread just enough on yourself to cover all exposed skin. Also spray it on clothing as well as tents, shoes, and other equipment you may be using. But don't use it *under* your clothing. You don't have to overdo it—extremely heavy amounts are not necessary to repel insects.

Protect your skin. Don't put repellant on cuts, wounds, or skin that is already irritated. The repellant can make an irritation worse. When you're back indoors, wash the repellant off with soap and water.

And your lungs. When you spray on repellant, do it in a well-ventilated area. You don't want to breathe it in. Don't pump or spray an aerosol in a closed-in area.

Keep repellant away from mucous membranes. Don't spray yourself in the face. The repellant might get in your eyes, where it can cause severe irritation. For your face: spray repellant on your hands, then rub it on; avoid getting it in your eyes or mouth.

Exercise caution with kids. Rub repellant on your own hands first and then put it on the children. Keep it out of kids' eyes and mouth. Don't put too much on their ears or any on their hands, as children frequently put their hands and fingers in their mouths. Never let kids under ten years of age put repellant on themselves, and store repellants in a safe area where they cannot reach them.

Newborns need netting. Infants less than two months old should not be exposed to DEET. Instead, protect them from mosquitoes with an infant carrier draped with mosquito netting. Use netting that has elastic borders so it fits tightly around the carrier.

Avoid peak periods. Stay indoors during twilight periods, at dawn or dusk, as well as at night in problem areas. Biting insects are most active and on the prowl at those times.

Cover up. Wear long pants, long-sleeved shirts, and hats to cover vulnerable areas of skin. Tuck your shirt in. For extra protection against insects, ticks, or chiggers, tuck your pants into your socks. Wear boots, never sandals.

Wear light-colored clothing. That makes it easier to spot ticks and insects you may have picked up. Frequently check yourself and your fellow travelers for ticks on your skin and clothing. If you take off a tick soon after it attaches, you lower your risk of infection.

Use adult bed nets at night. If the room you sleep in doesn't have screens or isn't shut up and air-conditioned, use bed nets to keep off mosquitoes and other insects. Bed nets should be treated with permethrin or another repellant. Permethrin acts as an effective repellant for several months if the net isn't washed. Tuck bed nets under mattresses. Before going to bed, consider using an aerosol insecticide to kill off mosquitoes that may already be in your bedroom.

Avoid combination products. Don't use products that combine repellant and sunscreen—sunscreen needs continual reapplication and that may mean overexposure to repellant.

Protect kids from ground dwellers. When children play on the soil where parasites are a risk, they should wear shoes or sneakers, not sandals. To minimize exposure to parasites, have the kids play on a towel, not right on the ground.

Your Gut Flush Traveling Health Kit

Especially if you find yourself traveling quite a bit, it's not a bad idea to take along a special travel kit, complete with all the Gut Flush supplements you'll need to be proactive against Colon Corruptors on the road. In addition, if you have particular allergies to medications or a health condition like diabetes, consider wearing an alert bracelet and an information card in your wallet or pocketbook that details what health care practitioners should know about you in case of emergency.

What to Put into Your Travel Kit

- Your Gut Flush Travel Kit supplements:
  - Your Gut Flush Basic Protocol (probiotics, HCl, and digestive enzymes)
  - Verma-Plus and Para-Key (A week before you leave on a trip, start taking the Verma-Plus and Para-Key products and continue during and after the conclusion of your trip for about three weeks.)
  - Extra supplies of probiotics in case of food poisoning (If you do get sick, take five of Dr. Ohhira's product every half hour until symptoms abate.)
  - Activated charcoal tablets to prevent and treat food poisoning (With

the activated charcoal, which can absorb food toxins and poisons, start with four capsules when the first symptoms appear, and use another four in one or two hours. Also, sprinkling some "chardust" on food can prevent problems.)

- Your prescription medications and copies of your prescriptions
- Antimalaria medicine if you're going to a malarial zone
- Cayenne pepper—helps with bronchitis, sore throat, as well as H. pylori and other Superbugs
- Arnica—homeopathic treatment for bruises; use cream for external application
- Bach Rescue Remedy—calming combination of flower essences that help you deal with traumatic situations and stress
- Dental floss—proper dental hygiene could prevent periodontal infections on the road
- Aloe vera gel—soothes sunburn or minor cuts
- Sunscreen—applied liberally and often
- Chamomile tea—an excellent relaxing brew for those anxious moments when luggage is lost or other traveling headaches hit (but make sure you make your tea with safe water!)
- Pau d'Arco and/or roasted dandelion root tea bags—antifungal and liver-protecting teas
- Ginger supplements—relieve motion sickness and helps digestion
- Insect repellant
- First-aid supplies like bandages, Ace wrapping, antiseptic ointment, tweezers, cotton swabs, scissors, and gauze.
- Small booklet that explains basic first-aid

Did You Bring Something Home?

Even with the best of precautions, if you pick up an infection or parasite while traveling, you may not know it right away. While some bugs make their presence known immediately, other problems may start to cause difficulties only weeks or months later (and some even take years!). Of course, the odds that you picked something up depends on where you traveled, how long you stayed, whether you followed good hygiene, and whether you already have compromised immunity.

If you do pick up a parasite or infection while traveling, usually you'll get symptoms within two weeks to two months or so. But an illness like malaria may take up to a year to make you ill. If you do become ill within twelve months of a trip, be sure to make your doctor aware of your trip. And if you develop a fever after going to a place where malaria is present, you need medical help for your condition immediately. If you think you might have malaria, you should be examined by a health practitioner who is experienced with tropical diseases. Even if your first lab tests seem to rule out malaria, you should have the tests repeated to make sure. You may need to be hospitalized.

When you develop a medical problem after traveling, tell your health care practitioner some key details: Did you go swimming in problem areas? Get insect bites? Animal bites? Did you eat raw food of any kind? Drink unpasteurized milk or dairy products? Did you have sexual contact during your trip? What kind of seafood did you eat? The answers to all of these questions can help pinpoint what your problem might be.

Depending on what happened during your trip, your physician may want to test your blood for malaria, do a blood cell count, check your liver enzymes, perform a chest X-ray, and culture your urine, blood, or stool samples (see Resources for parasite-certified testing labs).

If you need help finding a health care practitioner knowledgeable about tropical disease, consult the American Society of Tropical Medicine at http://www.astmh.org or the International Society of Travel Medicine at http://www.istm.org.

HOW LONG IT TAKES FOR TROPICAL DISEASES TO MAKE THEMSELVES KNOWN

Waiting Period	Symptoms	Possible Causes
< 2 weeks	Fever with initial nonspecific signs and symptoms	Malaria, chikungunya, dengue, scrub typhus, spotted group Rickettsiae, acute HIV, acute hepatitis C, *Campylobacter*, salmonellosis, shigellosis, East African trypanosomiasis, leptospirosis, relapsing fever, influenza, yellow fever
	Fever and excessive bleeding	Meningococcemia, leptospirosis, and other bacterial pathogens associated with coagulopathy, malaria, viral hemorrhagic fevers, enteroviruses
	Fever and central nervous system problems	Malaria, typhoid fever, rickettsial typhus (epidemic caused by *Rickettsia prowazecki*), meningococcal meningitis, rabies, arboviral encephalitis, East African trypanosomiasis, encephalitis or meningitis, angiostrongyliasis
	Fever and breathing difficulty	Influenza, pneumonia due to typical pathogens, *Legionella* pneumonia, acute histoplasmosis, acute coccidioidomycosis, Q fever, SARS
	Fever and skin rashes	Viral exanthems (rubella, measles, varicella, mumps, herpes simplex-6, enteroviruses) Chikungunya, dengue, spotted or typhus group rickettsiosis, typhoid fever, parvovirus B19
2 to 6 weeks	Fever with breathing problems, rashes, central nervous system difficulties, various other symptoms	Assorted illnesses: Malaria, tuberculosis, hepatitis A, hepatitis B, hepatitis C, hepatitis E, visceral leishmaniasis, acute schistosomiasis, amebic liver abscess, leptospirosis, African trypanosomiasis, viral hemorrhagic fevers, Q fever, acute American trypanosomiasis, viral causes of mononucleosis syndromes
> 6 weeks	Fever with breathing problems, rashes, central nervous system difficulties, various other symptoms	Assorted illnesses: Malaria, tuberculosis, hepatitis B, hepatitis E, visceral leishmaniasis, filariasis, onchocerciasis, schistosomiasis, amebic liver abscess, chronic mycoses, African trypanosomiasis, rabies, typhoid fever

Based on CDC Health Information for International Travel 2008;
http://wwwn.cdc.gov/travel/yellowBookCh2-PostTravel.aspx

Be Safe, Not Sorry, and Enjoy!

Let me repeat: Don't let all of this travel advice scare you from enjoying and exploring that wonderful world out there. Yes, more than ever, you do have to be aware of all the pitfalls and places where the Colon Corruptors may be lurking. But increased knowledge of the possible dangers empowers you to fight back. If you do get sick, you may more readily recognize the cause and possible cures so that you are your own best health advocate when working with a knowledgeable health practitioner. With common sense, preparation, and protection, you'll come home healthier and wiser about our global village.

16

Ensuring a Healthy Gut for Life

I'll admit it—we certainly face daunting health challenges in this day and age. No wonder we are becoming overwhelmed by the ever-increasing reports of MRSAs, parasites, fungi, bacteria, viruses, and food intolerances, the countless Colon Corruptors that are trying to gain a foothold in our bodies. But we have the wisdom—and now the tools—to do something about it, finally!

To use a popular buzzword from today's scientific world, I've designed the Gut Flush Plan for *sustainability*. If you follow the guidelines in the Gut Flush Plan to Fortify, Flush, and Feed your gut, to reduce your toxic load at home and on the road, and to be constantly vigilant for signs of Colon Corruptor infestation, you will keep yourself and your family safe from outside invaders. In addition, by continuing to follow all of these guidelines, you'll progressively enjoy better vitality, energy, and long-term, full-body health than you've ever experienced before. Perhaps most spiritually satisfying, by adhering to the principles I've laid out in this plan, you will automatically help to reduce certain toxic substances in the environment and support healthy agricultural practices that can ultimately help to heal our world.

Not bad for a deceptively delicious brand-new eating and lifestyle program, is it?

When I look to our future, in terms of gut health, I can't help but recall Dickens' famous quote, "It was the best of times, it was the worst of times, it was the age of wisdom, it was the age of foolishness." From my experience, that pretty much describes the situation we're in today. We continue to face a number of new and rising threats; but we can also see an equal number of exciting directions in research that point the way to powerful new solutions.

In conclusion, I want to acknowledge some of the emerging risks of Colon Corruptors in our Food Fright environment so that you will continue to stay on your toes and remain vigilant. I also want to take a moment to review some of the very exciting GI Good Guy developments coming down the pike. Despite a fair amount of evidence to the contrary, we are moving in the right direction—how long it takes everyone to catch up is another story. No matter what you or your family will face in the future, following the Gut Flush Plan will help keep you aware, strong, safe, and healthy, for life.

Emerging Challenges to Gut Health

Every day we learn about new and troubling fallout from new Colon Corruptors. For example, researchers are finding that there's a good chance some people may be obese because they are infected with certain viruses. In studies of twins, the heavier and fatter twin is more likely to show infection with a virus called Ad-36. This virus has also been shown to cause weight gain and obesity in chickens, mice, rats, and monkeys.

Signs are also popping up to suggest that we don't know the full extent of some risks already present in our environment. For instance, only recently a case of Chagas' disease, a parasitic infection passed on from an insect bite, was discovered in the United States. This illness, caused by the protozoan parasite Trypanosoma cruzi, is caught when you are bitten by so-called kissing bugs, and the infection itself can cause heart disease. But here's the scariest part: the infection can take *ten to twenty* years to develop. That means that we may have been exposed to Chagas' disease in this country for the last two decades, without any warning or any measures to prevent transfer and infection. Who knows how many similar parasites or other Colon Corruptors are lying dormant out there right now, let alone those that continue to develop?

Since forewarned is forearmed, the following information may help to save your life or that of a loved one someday—and perhaps, in the not so far distant future. Perhaps one of the most frightening parasites that could become a serious problem is the amoeba called Naegleria fowleri, reported to have killed about two dozen people in the United States between 1995 and 2004. The amoeba attacks the brain, entering through the nose; it thrives in warm water, and it is nearly always fatal. Researchers believe it lives in the mud at the bottom of swimming areas and may be stirred up into the water when people swim. More recently, people swimming in lakes and rivers in Florida, Texas, and Arizona have been overcome by this untreatable problem. As we continue to experience the effects of climate change, it is possible reports like this will become more common.

Meanwhile, as I've discussed throughout this book, antibiotic-resistant diseases also continue to rear their ugly heads. For instance, researchers now report that the parasite that causes river blindness is becoming resistant to ivermectin, the drug that has been used for about two decades to control this scourge. Ivermectin is considered the only safe drug for use to treat the 37 million people infected with Onchocerca volvulus, the parasitic nematode that causes river blindness. Researchers have called this discovery of a developing river-blindness Superbug a real wake-up call for figuring out new plans for controlling parasites.

You've heard how antibacterial soaps may be contributing to the creation of new Superbugs, but recent findings uncovered yet another reason we should avoid them. We now know that when the active ingredient in antibacterial soap, triclosan, is mixed with chlorinated tap water, chloroform vapor is released. Chloroform is a known carcinogen, and in its vapor form it can depress the response of humans' central nervous system, causing dizziness, fatigue, and unconsciousness. It's what's called a volatile organic compound, or VOC, a pollutant found in the air.

Along with toluene, benzene, and methyl tertiary butyl ether, chloroform is one of the four most common VOCs in our air. While other VOCs come from tobacco smoke, glue, shoe polish, and paint thinner, antibacterial cleaning products and air fresheners also produce large amounts of VOCs indoors. Researchers at the Johns Hopkins Bloomberg School of Public Health have recently discovered that the cancer risks from VOCs are much more serious than the Environmental Protection Agency (EPA) currently admits. And the Hopkins scientists found that EPA models showed only *one-third* of the toxic load that exists in reality.

Despite these shocking findings, triclosan continues to be added to all kinds of products. Because triclosan is so effective at killing bacteria, you can now find it in acne creams, lotions, hand soaps, dish soaps, cosmetics, and other personal care products. Manufacturers also add it to fabrics, medical devices, plastics, and polymers. Triclosan is even being used as a preservative in some foods.

I find all these new uses pretty worrisome. We haven't really studied the long-term effects of triclosan. Even the American Medical Association (AMA) has been on the FDA's case to look more closely at triclosan and other antimicrobials that we so blithely smear on our bodies. Every time you wash your hands or take a shower with an antibacterial soap, you're getting a good dose of chloroform—breathing it in and possibly absorbing it through your skin.

Oh, and did I mention the environmental effects of these soaps? Studies at the University of Minnesota demonstrate that when you wash triclosan down the drain, it goes into the environment and produces dioxin, another pollutant that wreaks havoc on the health of plants, animals, and humans.

Old-fashioned soap is looking better and better, right?

What concerns me about the future of our guts and the environment is that the profits of corporations are often considered more important than what their products do to our health.

Consider the case of air fresheners. The market for these products has exploded in the past decade. Particularly popular are the air fresheners that plug into the wall. Since 1989, when Glade invented the plug-in air freshener, sales of these odorous contraptions have soared until today the air freshener business has topped $4.5 billion.

What do we get for our $4.5 billion? According to researchers at the University of Washington, about one in five people have negative reactions to these devices. If you have asthma, you're in even bigger trouble—about a third of all the folks with asthma have trouble breathing and get headaches when inhaling an air freshener. The chemicals these things release—VOCs—cause allergic reactions and asthmatic attacks.

Sad to say, using an air freshener may superficially improve the smell of a house or room, but you're not getting to the root cause of the awful odor—you're merely covering it up with chemicals. So, if your house had mildew or mold—which can cause allergic reactions and contribute to gut problems and other illnesses—adding the VOCs of an air freshener only exacerbates the toxic burden your body has to bear. A better solution: clean up the damp parts of the house that are causing fungi to grow.

As scary as airborne VOCs are, countless toxins are considered permissible additives in the food supply—and when corporate profits are at stake, it's very hard to get them out. Consider the fact that in the year 2000, FDA regulators found that a pair of antibiotics fed to chickens had been conclusively tied to the development of antibiotic-resistant Superbugs in humans. In response, one pharmaceutical company rapidly recalled its drug, and farmers stopped giving it to poultry. But Bayer, the manufacturer of the other guilty drug, dragged the FDA to court to try to keep its drug on the market. It took *four years* of proceedings for a judge to finally tell Bayer to stop selling its drug (called Baytril) to farmers. But that didn't stop Bayer. It took another year for the drugmaker to finally drop its attempts to appeal the judge's decision.

This is just one example of how tough it is to clean up our diets and environment when big corporations *knowingly* make big profits from selling toxins. What happens when scientists are only just beginning to understand how certain food processes affect humans, even as those humans eat those foods?

The unknowns are a huge reason why I recommend against eating any genetically modified (GMO) foods. In my experience, these types of foods have introduced a whole new set of food allergies that we haven't even begun to understand. These alterations of foods have set in motion reactions to chemicals that traditionally have never been present in a wide range of foods. Animal genes have been inserted into plants, and plants have been changed to create unprecedented types of natural chemicals to which the human gut may never adapt—not to mention the devastating impact these genetic changes may make on our delicately balanced ecosystem.

Only by boycotting GMO foods and other dangerous products—such as air freshners, antibacterial cleaning products, other sources of VOCs—can we stop this kind of health and social destruction. Let's not allow our fear of bacteria to drive us to use products that work against our natural defenses. Let's not let the big corporations shortchange our health to fill their wallets. Instead, let's do what we can to work *with* our GI Good Guys and Fortify our bodies, Flush out invaders, and Feed ourselves and our GI systems well. And, thankfully, many researchers are working on ways for us to do just that.

New Directions in Gut Health

Fear not—there is hope for gut-healthier times! Mainstream science is now beginning to acknowledge the validity of many remedies that had previously been considered "fringe." Many strands of research are exploring how to use the GI Good Guys to support and defend our health. Perhaps the best example is the growing recognition of the power of probiotics.

Researchers in the United Kingdom have now shown that probiotics can fight Salmonella bacteria in pigs. They are actively working to have English pig farmers give their animals probiotics rather than antibiotics to fight infections and encourage better growth. It shocks me to realize that the Europeans are way ahead of us in this recognition—unlike the permissive United States, the European Union has now banned the use antibiotics in animal feed.

The British medical establishment is also out ahead of the United States in terms of using probiotics in humans. For example, a recent paper from the *British Medical Journal* showed a significant reduction of antibiotic-associated diarrhea in those who consumed a probiotic drink twice daily. And the researchers showed that the cost of using probiotics to mitigate antibiotic-associated diarrhea was just a fraction of the cost of treating it.

Slowly but surely, the tides are shifting in the United States as well. At a recent scientific meeting, Dr. Eamonn Quigley, vice president of the American College of Gastroenterology, explained the mechanism of immune activation and disruption of bacterial flora in irritable bowel syndrome (IBS). He showed that recent research is promising for specific probiotics in possibly reversing changes to the complex ecosystem of bacteria that live in the intestinal tract and affect the symptoms of IBS.

We know the power of probiotics to keep us healthy and to fight off Colon Corruptors. Every bit of research, each study that's released, all help to take probiotics into the mainstream awareness. It will be a happy day when probiotics supplements are as readily accepted and ingested as the humble daily vitamin.

Another topic that's gaining mainstream acceptance is the acknowledgment of the long-overlooked epidemic of celiac disease and gluten intolerance. As this awareness grows, researchers are drawing links between previously baffling health challenges and gluten sensitivity. Beyond relatively obvious intestinal symptoms—diarrhea, bloating, IBS symptoms—gluten sensitivity and celiac disease have been definitively linked to osteoporosis and weak bones, anemia, depression, and migraine headaches. Serious conditions such as colitis and diverticulis are also linked to gluten sensitivity. As part of the vicious cycle, Colon Corruptors are often to blame for causing these intolerances—damage to the intestines from Giardia may injure the intestinal walls and contribute to gluten intolerance and lactose intolerance.

Thankfully, everywhere you turn for nutrition information you can now find signs that awareness of the gluten sensitivity problem is growing. The National Institutes of Health (NIH) has created a celiac-awareness Web site for people who are sensitive to gluten (http://www.celiac.nih.gov). There are now special camps for kids that feature gluten-free menus, and at least three national support associations are available for those needing assistance. A search on Amazon.com for the word "gluten" yields a result of 10,170 books. You can even buy T-shirts, coffee mugs, and mouse pads that are designed to increase the awareness of gluten sensitivity. Whole Foods Market, the national chain of natural-organic supermarkets, now operates an 8,000-square-foot bakehouse in North Carolina devoted exclusively to producing gluten-free baked goods. By the year 2010, the market for gluten-free products is expected to edge close to $2 billion a year.

That's good news for all of us. Even if you don't have gluten sensitivity, you know that avoiding gluten gives any prospective Colon Corruptors less food to grow on. And as more and more people come to understand how certain foods and supplements can Fortify, Flush, and Feed the GI tract—and, above all, how good food and lifestyle choices support the GI Good Guys— the better, tastier, and healthier the entire food supply will become. As our bodies become stronger and the environment becomes cleaner, the less safe harbor we'll offer those Colon Corruptors. Perhaps we'll even see a day when the educated choices we make now will start to decimate their ranks, and we can return to a more idyllic time, before the rise of MRSA, antibiotic-laden meat, and the omnipresence of corn and gluten in our food supply.

For now, though, we must stand shoulder to shoulder to Fortify ourselves against Colon Corruptors' ranks—starting with what we put into our bodies every day.

That begins with the Gut Flush Plan.

The Gut Flush Plan for Life

You have in your hands all the information you need to start the Gut Flush Plan. I know these changes can be dramatic, but just keep your eye on the prizes. More energy. Less pain. Clear skin. Less anxiety and depression. Stronger bones. Bulletproof immunity. While you may consciously know that these benefits await you when you follow the Gut Flush Plan, I understand that it can sometimes be hard to stay on track. I offer these suggestions to help you maintain your motivation to take the steps necessary to revolutionize your health.

Stay informed. As the landscape of threats to gut health change, you have to recognize what new measures you have to take and what foods you must avoid. That means staying current with all the food scares that arise across the country—learn which foods are being recalled, which food additives are in the news, all about the latest research. One easy place to start is in the Resource section of this book. Also, regularly read the food and health pages of your local newspaper. Search the Internet by putting subjects like nutrition, probiotics, and health into search engines. Stay tuned in, and you'll learn about important scientific developments as they take place.

Pick a day to start the plan. And write it in red on your calendar. Research has shown that when people are considering making a change, moving from the "contemplation" stage to the "preparation" stage automatically makes them more likely to move to the "action" stage. As Goethe said, "Seize this very minute. . . . Boldness has genius, power and magic in it." Begin it now.

Turn off the television. Doing so will improve your chances of staying on the Gut Flush Plan. A slew of studies have shown that the more you watch

TV, the higher your chances of eating the junk food advertised so widely on TV shows. TV watchers also get less exercise and spend less time with their families at dinner and other group activities. TV may not be a Colon Corruptor, but it is certainly toxic!

Be faithful to your journal. Consistently writing in your journal about how much better you feel after you embark on the Gut Flush Plan can also reinforce your motivation for staying on the program. Put your feelings in writing. Make notes about the health difficulties you've had in the past and then describe how these have improved after you've paid more attention to what you eat, how much you exercise, and which supplements can help put you on the road to optimal health. Then you can periodically review your notes and use the improvements to keep your vigilance sharp.

Find a Gut Flush friend. Taking part in a buddy system is also a great way to stay on the program. Find somebody else who is also looking for a way

---

YOUR BLOOD, THE PARASITE FIGHTER

Exercise improves every aspect of health—it helps the gut function more effectively by simply encouraging waste products to move down and out. Exercise also boosts the immune system, helps to control weight, and lowers your risk of cancer. And by boosting your HDL (good cholesterol), exercise can also help your body ward off parasites.

Researchers have now conclusively shown that HDL is a key player in your body's antiparasite defenses. Scientists in Massachusetts have demonstrated that HDL takes part in your body's creation and delivery of two proteins that, when they combine, form a super-effective antimicrobial chemical. Although the scientists studied HDL's effect on a parasite called Trypanosoma brucei, an African nasty that gives animals a deadly disease known as nagana, this mechanism would likely work on many Colon Corruptors.

To get the maximum HDL benefit, be sure to pick up your pace and exert yourself. Aim for at least thirty to forty-five minutes of fast walking per day. That increase in exercise may help you fend off any parasites that threaten your well-being.

to improve their health. Share some research about the dangers of the conventional American diet and lifestyle. Really get each other's ire up. Then, join forces in fighting back. You can exercise together, cook together, and encourage each other. After a while, you may even want to organize your own Gut Flush Group that can share recipes, tips, and tricks on how to maintain the best Gut Health. I also invite you to come and visit www.annlouise.com/forum where you can get daily help 24/7 for any and all of your Gut Flush issues that relate to this book. There is a special section on the Forum for the Gut Flush Plan, especially devoted to you and your concerns.

Get your family involved. Get your husband or wife or kids to read this book. Talk to them about their health and their health issues to get them on the program. Expect some resistance. The marketing juggernaut that is the American food industry is geared up to convince us all that we deserve to have our health broken today by eating fast food, processed desserts, and snacks that drag our well-being down. Persist—for their sake, and for yours. If you can get your spouse involved in your new program, you increase your chances of success. (One study found that more than 90 percent of spouses who exercised together stuck to their program, but only about half of women who went it alone kept working out for a prolonged period of time.)

When you truly make up your mind to start the Gut Flush Plan, everything will fall into place. As you improve the health of your gut, as you Fortify, Flush, and Feed your system, you'll experience wonderful changes in your body and in your outlook in general. You'll know that you can face the future, and whatever it may hold, emboldened and strengthened by your greater confidence, energy, and vital health. Enjoy and be well!

Appendix
The Gut Flush Recipes

Cookery is not chemistry. It is an art. It requires instinct and taste.

—MARCEL BOULESTIN, chef

PROBIOTIC RECIPES

ANN LOUISE'S YOGURT

Here's that great probiotic food that can be used in so many ways and is delicious just by itself. You will need a food thermometer to accurately measure the temperature.

   1 quart milk (whole or 2 percent), organic if possible
   2 teaspoons Flora-Key OR 4 tablespoons store-bought yogurt with
      "live" cultures

Heat milk in a double boiler to 185–195 degrees F. Cool to about 130 degrees F. Add Flora-Key (see Resources) or store-bought yogurt. Pour into a 1-quart jar or 4 8-ounce jars with lids.

Place jar(s) in oven for 3–6 hours. If you use an electric oven, make sure the oven light is "on." This heated environment of about 110 degrees F. will allow the yogurt to "set." When yogurt is thickened, take out of oven and place directly in refrigerator.

MAKES FOUR 1-CUP SERVINGS

SIMPLE HOMEMADE SAUERKRAUT

If you've never tried to make your own sauerkraut, you are in for a treat. Crisp and tangy, this sauerkraut boasts natural enzymes and beneficial microflora in every bite.

   1 cup filtered water
   2 tablespoons lemon juice
   1 clove garlic, minced
   4 cups shredded cabbage (red and/or green)
   1 teaspoon dry mustard
   1 teaspoon caraway seeds
   1 teaspoon salt

In a small bowl, combine water, lemon juice, and garlic. In a 1-quart glass container with a cover, combine shredded cabbage, dry mustard, caraway seeds, and salt. Pour lemon juice mixture over cabbage.

Cover cabbage mixture tightly. Do not refrigerate. Keep at room temperature (no higher than 75 degrees F.) for at least three days, shaking occasionally. Fermentation usually begins in about a day.

MAKES I QUART OR FOUR I-CUP SERVINGS

MISO SOUP PLUS

For a richer mealtime soup, enjoy this version of miso for lunch or even try it for breakfast.

   2 tablespoons chopped shallots
   1 teaspoon minced fresh ginger
   ½ cup *each* thinly sliced cabbage and carrot
   1 teaspoon olive oil
   2 cups vegetable broth
   1 teaspoon almond butter
   2 tablespoons yellow miso
   2 tablespoons filtered water
   Minced chives, for garnish

In a medium saucepan, sauté shallots, ginger, and veggies in olive oil until crisp-tender, about 3 minutes. Add broth and almond butter and simmer gently for another 3–4 minutes. Dissolve miso in water and add to saucepan, stirring well.

Heat for another 5 minutes. *(Do not let soup boil.)* Top each serving with minced chives.

Store leftover soup in a covered container in the refrigerator.

MAKES THREE I-CUP SERVINGS

BAKED GOODIES

ALMOND MEAL MUFFINS

These protein-packed muffins are as healthy as they are delectable.

1 cup ground flaxseed
½ cup ground almonds or walnuts
¾ cup whey protein powder
½ teaspoon baking powder
1 teaspoon baking soda
1 teaspoon ground cinnamon
½ teaspoon ground cardamom
½ teaspoon salt
1 tablespoon coconut oil
2 eggs
2 teaspoons vanilla extract
⅔ cup grated carrot
⅔ cup soft tofu
Grated zest of 1 lemon

Preheat oven to 350 degrees F. Line a muffin tin with paper cups.

In a small bowl, mix ground flaxseed, ground nuts, whey protein powder, baking powder, baking soda, spices, and salt. In a large bowl, mix coconut oil, eggs, vanilla, grated carrot, tofu, and lemon zest. Fold dry ingredients into liquid ingredients, mixing until just combined. *Do not overmix.*

Pour mixture into prepared muffin tins and bake for 20–25 minutes, or until a wooden pick inserted into center of a muffin comes out clean and dry. *Do not overbake.*

Store leftover muffins in covered container in the refrigerator or freezer.

MAKES 6–8 MUFFINS (I MUFFIN PER SERVING)

MEGA-GRAIN QUICK BREAD

Try this for Sunday brunch and, if there are leftovers, next day's breakfast toast.

1 cup Montina gluten-free flour
1 cup quinoa flour
¼ cup ground flaxseed
½ cup sunflower seeds
¼ cup sesame seeds
½ teaspoon baking powder
½ teaspoon baking soda
½ teaspoon salt
⅓ cup coconut oil
2 eggs
1 cup unsweetened almond milk mixed with 1 tablespoon lemon juice
(Great buttermilk substitute!)

Preheat oven to 350 degrees F. Oil *bottom only* (bread will rise better) of one 9 x 5 x 3-inch loaf pans or two 8 x 4 x 2-inch loaf pans.

In a large bowl, mix flours, ground flaxseed, sunflower and sesame seeds, baking powder, baking soda, and salt. In a small bowl, stir together coconut oil, eggs, and almond milk mixture.

Pour liquid mixture over dry ingredients. Blend, but do not beat.

Spoon mixture into prepared pan and bake for 35–40 minutes, or until a wooden pick inserted in center comes out clean and dry. Place on cooling rack for about 10 minutes. Remove bread from pan; cool completely. Cut bread into 8 slices.

Store leftover bread in covered container in the refrigerator or freezer.

MAKES EIGHT 1-SLICE SERVINGS

ANN LOUISE'S TANGY TAPENADE

Serve this delicious and flavorful blend on grilled poultry, fish, or a burger, and, of course, with raw or steamed veggies.

2 tablespoons pitted black olives
2 tablespoons green olives with pimientos
2 tablespoons drained capers
¼ cup walnuts
½ cup fresh basil
2 garlic cloves, pressed
½ cup flaxseed oil
3 tablespoons fresh lemon juice
Salt and cayenne, to taste

Combine all ingredients in a food processor or electric blender, and pulse lightly to blend. Do not puree. Transfer to container with lid and refrigerate until serving time.

Store leftover tapenade in a covered container in the refrigerator.

MAKES I CUP OR FOUR ¼-CUP SERVINGS

GARBANZO BEAN HUMMUS

This quick and easy legume spread makes a fast snack or appetizer.

1 tablespoon *each* mint and cilantro
3 cloves garlic
1½ cups cooked dried garbanzo beans (chickpeas) OR 1 14.5-oz can
  garbanzo beans, rinsed and drained*
½ teaspoon salt
⅛ teaspoon cayenne

2 tablespoons olive oil
1 tablespoon lemon juice
1 teaspoon ground cumin

Pulse mint and cilantro with garlic in a food processor.

Add remaining ingredients and blend until smooth. Add a little water if needed until desired consistency is reached.

Store in a covered container in the refrigerator.

*If you have digestive issues, please use dry beans instead of canned beans.
How to Cook Dry Beans: www.centralbean.com/storeandsoak.html#Rinsing*

MAKES APPROXIMATELY 1½ CUPS OR SIX ¼-CUP SERVINGS

PARSLEY AND CILANTRO PESTO

This simple but intensely flavored pesto is a wonderful topping for vegetables, poultry, fish, and seafood. Oregano and garlic help keep those nasty Colon Corruptors at bay.

1½ cups *each* packed parsley and cilantro
2 teaspoons chopped oregano OR 1 teaspoon dried
3 cloves garlic
¼ cup pine nuts
1½ cups olive oil or flaxseed oil
¼ cup lemon juice

Place parsley, cilantro, oregano, garlic, pine nuts, and oil in a food processor or electric blender, and pulse until finely chopped. Add lemon juice, continuing to pulse until a paste forms, scraping down the sides as needed.

Store in a covered container in the refrigerator.

MAKES APPROXIMATELY 2 CUPS OR SIXTEEN 2-TABLESPOON SERVINGS

LEMON CAPER DRESSING

Lemony and loaded with healthy omega-3 fat, this dressing is great drizzled over grilled vegetables and bountiful garden salads.

½ cup flaxseed oil
¼ cup fresh lemon juice
2 tablespoons filtered water
2 teaspoons minced shallots
1 tablespoon lightly chopped capers
1 tablespoon chopped parsley
¼ teaspoon salt
Dash cayenne

Combine ingredients in a jar and shake well to mix.
Store in a covered container in the refrigerator.

MAKES I CUP OR EIGHT 2-TABLESPOON SERVINGS

MUST-HAVE MISO DRESSING

This simple recipe is terrific not only as a salad dressing but also as a marinade for seafood and chicken.

¼ cup lemon juice
1 tablespoon miso
1 small clove garlic, minced
3 tablespoons filtered water
2 tablespoons chopped chives
2 tablespoons flaxseed oil

Combine ingredients in a jar and shake well to mix.
Store in a covered container in the refrigerator.

MAKES ¾ CUP OR TWELVE 2-TABLESPOON SERVINGS

PARSLEY TAHINI SAUCE

This sesame-butter recipe is great on pasta and steamed vegetables, and also as a salad dressing.

2 cups parsley
1 cup tahini (sesame butter)
¼ cup lemon juice
½ cup filtered water
2 ounces soft tofu
½ teaspoon salt
1 teaspoon toasted sesame oil

Pulse parsley in a food processor until finely minced.

Add remaining ingredients; continue pulsing, adding a bit more water if needed until desired consistency is reached.

Store in a covered container in the refrigerator.

MAKES APPROXIMATELY 2 CUPS OR SIXTEEN 2-TABLESPOON SERVINGS

RANCH DRESSING

This new and improved version will surprise you with its zesty flavors.

1 cup Vegenaise
¼ cup plain yogurt
⅓ cup fresh lime juice
1 teaspoon minced garlic
1 tablespoon minced shallot
½ teaspoon salt
¼ teaspoon cayenne pepper
½ teaspoon each chopped parsley, basil, and cilantro

Combine all ingredients in a jar and shake well to mix.

Store in a covered container in the refrigerator.

MAKES 1½ CUPS OR TWELVE 2-TABLESPOON SERVINGS

QUINOA TABBOULI

This twist on a popular Middle Eastern favorite is perfect for lunches or as a quick snack. Add more lemon juice if you prefer a little extra zip.

1 cup uncooked quinoa
1 teaspoon salt
⅓ cup chopped pumpkin seeds (toasted, if desired)
1 medium cucumber, seeded and chopped
½ cup chopped parsley
2 tablespoons chopped mint
1 cup cherry tomatoes, quartered OR 2 plum tomatoes, chopped
2 tablespoons flaxseed oil
2–3 tablespoons lemon juice
Salt, to taste
Cayenne, to taste

Place quinoa in a small-meshed strainer; rinse and drain well. Place drained quinoa in a medium skillet over low heat; toast for about 5 minutes, shaking pan occasionally. In a medium saucepan, bring 2 cups of water to a boil; add toasted quinoa and salt. Return to a boil; reduce heat and simmer, covered, for 20 minutes. Fluff with a fork. Let cool for about 20 minutes.

In a large bowl, toss quinoa with remaining ingredients. Let stand for about 15 minutes before serving to allow flavors to "meld," or refrigerate for later use.

Store leftover tabbouli in a covered container in the refrigerator.

MAKES 4 CUPS OR FOUR I-CUP SERVINGS

MAIN COURSES

■

AMARANTH-AND-HERB-CRUSTED CHICKEN

Equally suitable for a quick midweek or company dinner, this dish makes a lovely presentation. Amaranth is a wonderful choice for gluten-free breading.

¼ cup pine nuts, for garnish
½ cup pine nuts, ground

1 cup puffed amaranth cereal, ground
⅛ teaspoon salt
¼ cup Vegenaise
2 teaspoons Dijon mustard
2 tablespoons *each* minced oregano and parsley
¼ teaspoon red pepper flakes
6 organic boneless, skinless chicken breast halves (5 oz each)
1 tablespoon olive oil
Juice of 1 lemon
Minced parsley, for garnish

Preheat oven to 375 degrees F. Toast pine nuts in a dry skillet over low heat till lightly browned; set aside. Lightly coat a 9 x 13-inch baking dish with olive oil spray.

In a shallow baking dish, combine toasted ground pine nuts, ground amaranth, and salt. In a medium bowl, combine Vegenaise, Dijon mustard, oregano, parsley, and red pepper flakes. Coat both sides of chicken in Vegenaise mixture followed by ground amaranth–pine nut mixture. Arrange chicken in prepared baking dish; drizzle with olive oil and lemon juice.

Bake for approximately 40 minutes, or until chicken reaches 165 F. degrees on meat thermometer. Remove from oven and top with remaining toasted pine nuts and minced parsley.

Note: Freeze leftover chicken breasts for easy on-the-go meals.

MAKES 6 SERVINGS

TURKEY MEAT LOAF FLORENTINE

Not only is this meat loaf hearty and filling, it makes a lovely presentation on guests' dinner plates.

½ cup + 3 tablespoons marinara sauce, divided
1 10-oz package frozen chopped spinach, thawed and squeezed dry
1 medium onion, chopped
2 cloves garlic, minced
½ lb ground white turkey breast

½ lb ground dark turkey meat
¾ cup rolled oats
1 large egg
1 teaspoon salt
Dash cayenne
1 teaspoon *each* dried sage and rosemary
1½ teaspoons Dijon mustard
Fresh parsley, for garnish

Preheat oven to 350 degrees F. Mix 3 tablespoons marinara sauce and squeezed-dry spinach; set aside. In a small skillet, sauté onion and garlic until lightly browned. Place white and dark ground turkey in a large bowl. Pulse oats in a food processor or electric blender until finely ground. Add the onion mixture, egg, salt, cayenne, herbs, and mustard and mix well.

Line a baking sheet with parchment paper. Place turkey mixture onto prepared sheet; pat into a 14 x 10-inch rectangle. Layer spinach-marinara sauce combination over turkey mixture, spreading until it reaches within ¾ inch of edges on all sides. Beginning at short end, roll up jelly-roll fashion, pinching ends closed.

Bake for 40 minutes. Spread remaining ½ cup marinara sauce over the top of meat loaf and bake an additional 10 minutes, or until a meat thermometer reads 160 degrees F. Cool slightly; slice. Garnish with parsley.

Note: Leftover meat loaf freezes well.

MAKES 6 4-OUNCE SERVINGS

SOUPS

CREAMY KABOCHA SQUASH SOUP

Another sweet and meaty squash, such as delicata or butternut, can be used in this simple, vitamin A–rich soup.

1 medium kabocha squash
1 cup chopped onion
2 large cloves garlic

¼ cup olive oil

3 cups chicken broth, divided

1 teaspoon salt

½ teaspoon ground turmeric

¼ cup chopped parsley

¼ teaspoon ground nutmeg

Preheat oven to 375 degrees F. Lightly coat a baking dish with olive oil spray. Cut squash in half, leaving in seeds; place cut side down in baking dish.

Bake for approximately 45 minutes, or until very soft. Cool.

In a large saucepan, sauté onion and garlic in olive oil over medium heat until soft.

Deglaze the pan with 1 cup chicken broth; add salt and simmer another 15 minutes.

Remove seeds from squash and scoop the cooked squash into a food processor or electric blender. Add onion, garlic, and broth mixture and puree until smooth.

Return puree to saucepan, add remaining chicken broth, and gently simmer for another 10 minutes. Stir in turmeric, parsley, and nutmeg just before serving (adding these seasonings last preserves color and inhibits bitterness).

Store leftover soup in a covered container in the refrigerator.

MAKES I QUART OR FOUR I-CUP SERVINGS

QUICK AND EASY CARROT SOUP

This satisfying soup is rich in color and vitamin A.

3 cups chicken broth

1½ cups coarsely chopped carrots

¼ cup chopped shallots

1 tablespoon chopped garlic

1 teaspoon salt

2 teaspoons flaxseed oil

2 teaspoons lemon juice

Combine all ingredients except flaxseed oil and lemon juice in a medium saucepan; simmer until carrots are tender, about 20 minutes. Puree mixture in a food processor or electric blender. Ladle into bowls; drizzle with flaxseed oil and lemon juice.

Store leftover soup in a covered container in the refrigerator.

MAKES I QUART OR FOUR I-CUP SERVINGS

SAVORY TURKEY AND SWISS CHARD SOUP

A zippy one-pot meal, this soup is delicious served with a salad on a weeknight and again for next day's lunch.

½ cup sliced red onion
2 cloves garlic, minced
2 teaspoons olive oil
4 cups chicken broth
1 cup diced turkey breast (about 6 oz)
½ teaspoon *each* dried sage, thyme, and parsley
⅛ teaspoon red pepper flakes
1 bay leaf
4 cups sliced Swiss chard
1 14.5-oz can crushed tomatoes
2 tablespoons lemon juice
½ teaspoon salt

In a 2-quart saucepan, sauté onion and garlic in olive oil until soft.

Add the chicken broth, turkey, herbs, pepper flakes, and bay leaf. Simmer for 15 minutes.

Remove bay leaf; add Swiss chard, tomatoes, lemon juice, and salt.

Continue to simmer for another 10 minutes, until chard wilts.

Store leftover soup in a covered container in the refrigerator.

MAKES 2 QUARTS OR EIGHT I-CUP SERVINGS

BLACK BEAN 'N' BEEF CHILI WITH A TWIST

Power-packed with fiber, this colorful hearty dish will please your entire family.

1 tablespoon olive oil, divided
2 cloves garlic, minced
1 onion, chopped
1 lb lean ground beef
1 zucchini, sliced lengthwise and quartered
2 carrots, sliced
1 small head red cabbage, coarsely chopped
1½ cups cooked dried black beans* OR 1 14.5-oz can black beans,
    rinsed and drained
1 28-oz can crushed tomatoes
1 14-oz can diced tomatoes
2 tablespoons tomato paste
2 teaspoons *each* oregano, cumin, and chili powder
½ teaspoon salt
Cayenne, to taste
¼ cup *each* chopped parsley and cilantro
Chopped parsley and cilantro, for garnish

In a large skillet, heat 1 teaspoon olive oil over medium-high heat.
Sauté garlic and onion with ground beef until cooked through; drain. Remove to a bowl. Heat remaining 2 teaspoons olive oil over medium-high
heat. Add vegetables, sautéeing until crisp-tender. Stir in black beans,
crushed and diced tomatoes, tomato paste, reserved beef and onion mixture,
and seasonings. Bring to a boil; reduce heat, cover, and simmer for about 20
minutes. Stir in chopped parsley and cilantro. Ladle into bowls; top with
additional chopped parsley and cilantro, as desired.

If you have digestive issues, please use dry beans instead of canned beans.
How to Cook Dry Beans: www.centralbean.com/storeandsoak.html#Rinsing.

MAKES 4 SERVINGS OF APPROXIMATELY 2 CUPS EACH

Source Notes

Introduction

1. Puschner, B. "Assessment of melamine and cyanuric acid toxicity in cats." *J Vet Diagn Invest.* 2007 Nov.; 19(6): 616–24
2. Mead, P. S. "Food Related Death and Illness in the United States, Emerging Infectious Diseases." Vol. 5, #5; www.cdc.gov/ncidod/eid/vol5no5/mead.htm#1
3. Weiss, Rick. "Tainted Chinese Imports Common." *Washington Post,* 5/20/07.
4. Klevens, R. M. "Invasive Methicillin-Resistant Staphylococcus Infections in the United States," *JAMA.* 2007; 298: 1763–1777.

Chapter 1

1. Graves E. J., Gillium B. S. "Detailed diagnoses and procedures, National Hospital Discharge Survey, 1995." National Center for Health Statistics. *Vital Health Stat* 1997; 13.
2. 1998 FoodNet Surveillance Results. Preliminary Report. Atlanta: Centers for Disease Control and Prevention; 1999.
3. Mead, P. S. "Food Related Death and Illness in the United States, Emerging Infectious Diseases." Vol. 5, #5; www.cdc.gov/ncidod/eid/vol5no5/mead.htm#1
4. Dunkley, K. D. "Growth and genetic responses of Salmonella typhimurium to pH-shifts in an anaerobic continuous culture." *Anaerobe.* 11/29/07.
5. "Demographics Boon to Laxatives," *Chain Drug Review.* 1/3/94.

6. "Constipation," NIH Publication No. 07–2754. July 2007. http://digestive .niddk.nih.gov/ddiseases/pubs/constipation

7. Shen, E. P. "The Changing Face of Clostridium Difficile: What Treatment Options Remain?" *Am J Gastroenterol.* 2007 Dec.; 102(12): 2789–92.

8. Zaidi, E. "CT and clinical features of acute diverticulitis in an urban U.S. population: rising frequency in young, obese adults." *AJR Am J Roentgenol.* 2006 Sept.; 187(3): 689–94.

9. Shaheen, N. J. "The burden of gastrointestinal and liver diseases, 2006." *Am J Gastroenterol.* 2006 Sept.; 101(9):2128–38.

10. Yang, Y. "Long-term Proton Pump Inhibitor Therapy and Risk of Hip Fracture." *JAMA.* 2006; 296:2947–2953.

11. Boyette, K. "The medical masquerader." *J Miss State Med Assoc.* 2007 March; 48(3): 72–6.

12. Chey, W. D. "Guidelines on the Management of Helicobacter pylori infection." *Am J Gastroenterol.* 2007; 102: 1808–1825.

Chapter 2

1. Zavros, Y. "Hypergastrinemia in response to gastric inflammation suppresses somatostatin." *Am J Physiol Gastrointest Liver Physiol.* 282: G175–G183, 2002.

2. Lipski, Elizabeth. *Digestive Wellness* (McGraw-Hill, 2004), pg. 191.

3. Huffnagle, Gary B. *The Probiotics Revolution* (Bantam, 2007), pp. 80–82.

4. Alfredson, D. A. "Antibiotic resistance and resistance mechanisms in Campylobacter jejuni and Campylobacter coli." *FEMS Microbiol Lett.* 2007 Dec; 277(2): 123–32.

5. Wenzel, R. P. "Clinical practice. Acute bronchitis." *N Engl J Med.* 2006 Nov. 16; 355(20): 2125–30.

6. Huffnagle, op. cit., p. 326.

7. Lopez, D.A. *Enzymes, the Fountain of Life* (Neville Press, 1994), pp. 103–13.

8. Takai, N. "Effect of psychological stress on the salivary cortisol and amylase levels in healthy young adults." *Psychoneuroendorcinology.* 2006 Jan.; 31(1): 49–58.

Chapter 3

1. Huffnagle, Gary B. *The Probiotics Revolution* (Bantam, 2007), pg. 30.

2. Bahn, Y. S. "CAP1, an Adenylate Cyclase-Associated Protein Gene, Regulates Bud-Hypha Transitions, Filamentous Growth, and Cyclic AMP Levels and Is Required for Virulence of Candida Albicans." *J Bacteriol.* 2001 May; 183(10): 3211–3223.

3. Kennedy, M. J. "Effect of various antibiotics on gastrointestinal colonization and dissemination by Candida." *Medical Mycology.* Vol. 23, Issue 41985, pp. 265–273.

4. Yakai, S. "Candida boidinii peroxisomal membrane protein Pmp30 has a role in

peroxisomal proliferation and is functionally homologous to Pmp27 from Saccharomyces cerevisiae." *J Bacteriol.* 1995 Dec.; 177(23): 6773–6778.

5. Shoubridge, E. A. "The human cytochrome c oxidase assembly factors SCO1 and SCO2 have regulatory roles in the maintenance of cellular copper homeostasis." *Cell Metab.* 2007 Jan; 5(1):9–20. Erratum in: *Cell Metab.* 2007 May; 5(5): 403.
6. Crook, William. *The Yeast Connection* (Vintage, 1986).
7. Al Waili, N. S. "Effects of heating, storage and ultraviolet exposure on antimicrobial activity of garlic juice." *Jrnl Food Med.* 2007 March; 10(1): 208–12.
8. Adeleye, I. A. "Antimicrobial activity of extracts of local cough mixtures on upper respiratory tract bacterial pathogens." *West Indian Med J.* 2003 Sept.; 52(3): 188–90.
9. Galland, Leo. *The Four Pillars of Healing* (Random House, 1997).
10. Valnet, Jean. *The Practice of Aromatherapy* (Inner Traditions, 1990), pg. 34.

Chapter 4

1. MacKenzie, W. R. "A Massive Outbreak in Milwaukee of Cryptosporidium Infection Transmitted Through the Public Water Supply." *NEJM.* Vol. 331: 161–167.
2. Bern, C. "Epidemiologic Studies of Cyclospora cayetanensis in Guatemala." *Emerging Infectious Diseases.* Vol. 5, No. 6 / November–December 1999.
3. Schilder, R. J., "Metabolic syndrome and obesity in an insect." *PNAS, USA.* 2006 Dec. 5; 103(49): 18805–9.
4. Stanley, S. L., R. J. Jr. "Amoebiasis." *Lancet,* 2003 March; 22; 361(9362): 1025–34.
5. Halstead, S. B. "Dengue." *Lancet.* 2007 Nov; 10; 370(9599): 1644–52.
6. Hemmer C. J. "Global warming: trailblazer for tropical infections in Germany?" *Dtsch Med Wochenschr.* 2007 Nov.; 132(48): 2583–9.
7. Powell, J. "ConAgra Hamburger Recall Is Nation's Second Largest." *Star Tribune,* 2002.
8. Hennessy, T. W., Hedberg, C. W., Slutsker, L., White, K. E., Besser-Wiek. J. M., Moen. M. E. et al. "A national outbreak of Salmonella enteridis infection from ice cream." *N Engl J Med.* 1996; 334: 1281–6.
9. Centers for Disease Control and Prevention. "Outbreaks of Shigella sonnei infection associated with eating fresh parsley—United States and Canada, July–August 1988." *MMWR Morb Mortal Wkly Rep.* 1999; 48: 285–9.
10. Fischer, A. R. "Food safety in the domestic environment: an interdisciplinary investigation of microbial hazards during food preparation." *Risk Anal.* 2007 Aug.; 27(4): 1065–82.
11. Deardorff, T. L. "Invasive anisakiasis. A case report from Hawaii." *Gastroenterology.* 1986 April; 90(4): 1047–50.
12. Thompson, R. C. "The public health and clinical significance of Giardia and Cryptosporidium in domestic animals." *Vet J.* 2007 Nov. 19.

13. Curtis, V. "Effect of washing hands with soap on diarrhea risk in the community: a systematic review." *The Lancet Infectious Diseases,* Vol. 3, Issue 5, pp. 275–81.
14. Webb, A. L. "Update: effects of antioxidant and nonantioxidant vitamin supplementation on immune function." *Nutr Rev.* 2007 May; 65(5): 181–217.
15. Maggini, S. "Selected vitamins and trace elements support immune function by strengthening epithelial barriers and cellular and humoral immune responses." *Br J Nutr.* 2007 Oct.; 98 Suppl 1:S29–35.
16. Shin, S. Y. "Antibacterial activity of bioconverted eicosapentaenoic (EPA) and docosahexaenoic acid (DHA) against foodborne pathogenic bacteria." *Intl Jrnl Food Microbio.* 2007 Jan. 25; 113(2): 233–6.
17. Agarwal, V. "Prevention of Candida albicans biofilm by plant oils *Mycopathologia.*" 2007 Oct. 30.
18. Vidal. F. "Giardia lamblia: the effects of extracts and fractions from Mentha x piperita Lin. (Lamiaceae) on trophozoites." *Exp Parasitol.* 2007 Jan.; 115(1): 25–31.

Chapter 5

1. Klevins, R. N. "Invasive Methicillin–Resistant Staphylococcus Aureus Infections in the United States." *JAMA.* 2007; 298: 1763–1771.
2. "The growing threat of foodborne bacterial enteropathogens of animal origin." *Clin Infect Dis.* 2007 Nov. 15; 45(10): 1353–61.
3. Centers for Disease Control and Prevention. "Preliminary FoodNet data on the incidence of infection with pathogens transmitted commonly through food—10 states." *MMWR Morb Mortal Wkly Rep.* 2007 April 13; 56(14): 336–9.
4. Centers for Disease Control and Prevention. "Turtle–associated salmonellosis in humans—United States, 2006–2007." *MMWR Morb Mortal Wkly Rep.* 2007 July 6; 56(26): 649–52.
5. Kassenborg, H. D. "Farm visits and undercooked hamburgers as major risk factors for sporadic Escherichia coli O157:H7 infection: data from a case-control study in 5 FoodNet sites." *Clin Infect Dis.* 2004 April 15; 38 Suppl 3: S271–8.
6. Tuttle, J. "Lessons from a large outbreak of Escherichia coli O157:H7 infections: insights into the infectious dose and method of widespread contamination of hamburger patties." *Epidemiol Infect.* 1999 April; 122(2): 185–92.
7. Serna, A. IV, "Pathogenesis and treatment of Shiga toxin–producing Escherichia coli infections." *Curr Opin Gastroenterol.* 2008 Jan.; 24(1): 38–47.
8. McCaskil, M. L. "Increase of the USA300 clone among community-acquired methicillin-susceptible Staphylococcus aureus causing invasive infection." *Pediatr Infect Dis J.* 2007 Dec.; 26(12):1122–7.
9. Bogdanovich, T. "Genetic characterization of erythromycin- and methicillin-resistant community-acquired Staphylococcus aureus isolated from children in Texas." *Diagn Microbiol Infect Dis.* 2007 Oct.; 59(2): 231–3.

10. Chey, W. D. "American College of Gastroenterology guideline on the management of Helicobacter pylori infection." *Am J Gastroenterol,* 2007 Aug.; 102: 1808–1825.

11. Stettin, D. "Infection with Helicobacter pylori—outcome of a cross-sectional investigation." *Dtsch Med Wochenschr.* 2007 Dec.; 132(50): 2677–82.

12. Naous, A. "Fecoprevalence and determinants of Helicobacter pylori infection among asymptomatic children in Lebanon." *J Med Liban.* 2007 July–Sept.; 55(3): 138–44.

13. Poms, R. E. "Survival of H. pylori in ready-to-eat foods at 4 degrees C." *Intl Jrnl Food Microbio.* 2001 Feb. 15; 63(3): 281–6.

14. Davies, Lawrence E. "Businessmen Get Advice on Ulcers." *New York Times,* 4/5/60.

15. Roelofs, C. "Results from a Community-based Occupational Health Survey of Vietnamese-American Nail Salon Workers." *J Immigr Minor Health.* 2007 Oct. 18.

16. Fahey, J. W. "Sulforaphane inhibits extracellular, intracellular, and antibiotic-resistant strains of Helicobacter pylori and prevents benzo[a]pyrene-induced stomach tumors." *Proc Natl Acad Sci USA.* 2002 May 28; 99(11): 7610–5.

17. Lee, I. O. "Anti–inflammatory effect of capsaicin in Helicobacter pylori–infected gastric epithelial cells." *Helicobacter.* 2007 Oct; 12(5): 510–7.

18. Siddaraju, M. N. "Inhibition of gastric H(+),K(+)-ATPase and Helicobacter pylori growth by phenolic antioxidants of Curcuma amada." *J Agric Food Chem.* 2007 Sept. 5; 55(18): 7377–86.

19. Paraschos, S. "In vitro and in vivo activities of Chios mastic gum extracts and constituents against Helicobacter pylori." *Antimicrob Agents Chemother.* 2007 Feb.; 51(2): 551–9.

20. Lv, R. L. "The effects of aloe extract on nitric oxide and endothelial levels in deep-partial thickness burn wound tissue in rat." *Zhonghua Shao Shang Za Zhi.* 2006 Oct.; 22(5): 362–5.

21. Vogler, B. K. "Aloe Vera, a systematic review of its clinical effectiveness." *Brit Jrnl Gen Prac.* 1999 Oct.; 49(447): 823–8.

Chapter 6

1. Smith, Melissa Diane. *Going Against the Grain* (Contemporary Books, 2002), pp. 88–91.

2. Gaeta, T. J. "National study of US emergency department visits for acute allergic reactions, 1993 to 2004." *Ann Allergy Asthma Immunol.* 2007 April; 98(4): 360–5.

3. Shurin, M. R. "Immune-mediated diseases: where do we stand?" *Adv Exp Med Biol.* 2007; 601: 3–12. Review

4. Burks, W. "Current Understanding of Food Allergy." *Ann NY Acad Sci.* 2002 May; 964: 1–12.

5. Samson, K. T. "IgE binding to raw and boiled shrimp proteins in atopic and nonatopic patients with adverse reactions to shrimp." *Intl Arch Allergy Immunol.* 2004 March; 133(3): 225–32.

6. Droste, J. H. "Does the use of antibiotics in early childhood increase the risk of asthma and allergic disease?" *Clin Exp Allergy.* 2000 Nov.; 30(11): 1547–53.

7. Lomer, M. C. "Review article: lactose intolerance in clinical practice—myths and realities." *Aliment Pharmacol Ther.* 2007 Oct. 23.

8. Yang, W. H. "The monosodium glutamate symptom complex: assessment in a double-blind, placebo-controlled, randomized study." *Jrnl Allergy Clin Immunol.* 1997 June; 99(6 Pt 1): 757–62.

9. Egger, J. "Controlled trial of oligoantigenic treatment in the hyperkinetic syndrome." *Lancet.* 1985 March 9; 1(8428): 540–5.

10. Underwood, Ann. "Waiter, Please Hold the Wheat." *Newsweek.* 9/17/07.

11. Fasano, A. "Prevalence of celiac disease in at-risk and not-at-risk groups in the United States: a large multicenter study." *Arch Intern Med.* 2003 Feb. 10; 163(3): 286–92.

12. Hu, W. T. "Cognitive impairment and celiac disease." *Archives of Neurology.* 2006 Oct.; 63(10): 1440–6.

13. Dolinsek, J. "The prevalence of celiac disease among family members of celiac disease patients." *Wien Klin Wochenschr.* 2004; 116 Suppl 2: 8–12.

14. Sheiner, E. "Pregnancy outcome of patients with known celiac disease." *Eur Jrnl Obstet Gyn Reprod Biol.* 2006 Nov.; 129(1): 41–5.

15. Prescott, J. "Does information about MSG content influence consumer ratings of soups with and without added MSG?" *Appetite.* 2002 Aug.; 39(1): 25–33.

16. Calder, P. C. "Immunomodulation by omega-3 fatty acids." *Prostaglandins Leukot Essent Fatty Acids.* 2007 Nov.–Dec.; 77(5–6): 327–35.

Chapter 7

1. http://www.mnwelldir.org/docs/history/biographies/louis_pasteur.htm

2. Huffnagle, Gary. *The Probiotics Revolution* (Bantam, 2007), pg. 5.

3. De Preter, V., Coopmans, T., Rutgeerts, P., Verbeke, K. "Influence of long-term administration of lactulose and Saccharomyces boulardii on the colonic generation of phenolic compounds in healthy human subjects." *J Am Coll Nutr.* 2006 Dec.; 25(6): 541–9.

4. Huffnagle, op. cit. pg. 103.

5. Metchnikoff, Elie. *Immunity in Infective Diseases* (Cambridge University Press, 1907), pg. 430.

6. *Women's Health Newsletter,* Oct. 2004.

7. Gibson, G. R. "Dietary modulation of the human gut microflora using prebiotics." *Brit Jrnl Nutr,* 1998 Oct.; 80(4): S209–12.

8. Abrams, S. A. "A combination of prebiotic short- and long-chain inulin type fructans enhances calcium absorption." *Am J Clin Nutr.* Vol. 82, No. 2, 471–476, August 2005.

9. Waldecker, M. "Inhibition of histone deacetylase activity by short-chain fatty acids." *Jrnl N Biochem.* 11/29/07.

10. Calder, P. C. "Immunomodulation by omega-3 fatty acids." *Prostaglandins Leukot Essent Fatty Acids.* 2007 Nov.–Dec.; 77(5–6): 327–35.

11. Shin, S. Y. "Antibacterial activity of bioconverted eicosapentaenoic (EPA) and docosahexaenoic acid (DHA) against foodborne pathogenic bacteria." *Int Jrnl Food Microbio.* 2007 Jan. 25; 113(2): 233–6.

12. McKay, D. L. "A review of the bioactivity of South African herbal teas." *Phytother Res* 2007 Jan.; 21(1): 1–16.

13. Pedersen, M. "Strong combined gene-environment effects in anti-cyclic citrullinated peptide-positive rheumatoid arthritis." *Arthritis Rheum.* 2007 May; 56(5): 1446–53.

14. Sile, S. "Functional BSND variants in essential hypertension." *Am J Hypertens.* 2007 Nov.; 20(11): 1176–1182.

Chapter 8

1. Johanson, J. F. "Review of the treatment options for chronic constipation." *MedGenMed.* 2007 May 2; 9(2): 25.

2. Watzl, B. "Modulation of human T-lymphocyte functions by the consumption of carotenoid-rich vegetables." *Brit Jrnl Nutr.* 1999 Nov.; 82(5): 383–9.

3. Waitzberg, D. L. "New parenteral lipid emulsions for clinical use." *JPEN.* 2006 July–Aug.; 30(4): 351–67.

4. Lopez, V. "In vitro antioxidant and anti–rhizopus activities of Lamiaceae herbal extracts." *Plant Foods Hum Nutr.* 2007 Dec.; 62(4): 151–5.

5. Smith, Melissa Diane. *Going Against the Grain* (Contemporary Books, 2002), pg. 181.

Chapter 9

1. Cash, H. L. "Symbiotic bacteria direct expression of an intestinal bactericidal lectin." *Science.* 2006 Aug 25; 313(5790): 1126–30.

2. Noakes, M. "Effect of an energy-restricted, high-protein, low-fat diet relative to a conventional high-carbohydrate, low-fat diet on weight loss, body composition, nutritional status, and markers of cardiovascular health in obese women." *Am J Clin Nutr.* 2005 June; 81(6): 1298–1306

3. Attaix, D. "Altered responses in skeletal muscle protein turnover during aging in anabolic and catabolic periods." *Int J Biochem Cell Biol.* 2005 Oct.; 37(10): 1962–73.

4. Layman, D. K. "A reduced ratio of dietary carbohydrate to protein improves body composition and blood lipid profiles during weight loss in adult women." *J Nutr.* 2003 Feb.; 133(2): 411–17.

5. Didier, R. "Postprandial whole-body protein metabolism after a meat meal is influenced by chewing efficiency in elderly subjects." *Am J Clin Nutr.* 2007 May; 85: 1286–92.

6. Sherman, P. W. "Why vegetable recipes are not very spicy." *Evol Hum Behav.* 2001 May; 22(3): 147–63.

7. Zhang, L. "Intestinal and hepatic glucuronidation of flavonoids." *Mol Pharm.* 2007 Nov.–Dec.; 4(6): 833–45.

8. Scanlon Cunha, L. C. "Antibacterial activity of triterpene acids and semi–synthetic derivatives against oral pathogens." *Z Naturforsch* [C]. 2007 Sept.–Oct.; 62(9–10): 668–72.

9. Muller, T. "Colorless tetrapyrrolic chlorophyll catabolites found in ripening fruit are effective antioxidants." *Angew Chem Int Ed Engl.* 2007; 46(45): 8699–8702.

10. Dewanto, V. "Thermal processing enhances the nutritional value of tomatoes by increasing total antioxidant activity." *J Agric Food Chem.* 2002 May 8; 50(10): 3010–14.

11. Bednar, G. E. "Starch and fiber fractions in selected food and feed ingredients affect their small intestinal digestibility and fermentability and their large bowel fermentability in vitro in a canine model." *J Nutr.* 2001 Feb.; 131(2): 276–86.

12. Sampathkumar, S. G. "Targeting glycosylation pathways and the cell cycle: sugar-dependent activity of butyrate-carbohydrate cancer prodrugs." *Chem Biol.* 2006 Dec.; 13(12): 1265–75.

13. Duke, J. A. *Dr. Duke's Phytochemical and Ethnobotanical Databases.* Agricultural Research Service (ARS), Phytochemical Database, USDA. Beltsville Agricultural Research Center, Beltsville, Md. http://www.ars–grin.gov/cgi–bin/duke/ethnobot.pl

14. University of Maryland Medical Center Alternative Medicine Database. http://www.umm.edu/altmed/articles/slippery-elm-000274.htm

15. Li, J. "Glutamine prevents parenteral nutrition-induced increases in intestinal permeability." *J Parenter Interal Nutr.* 1994 July-Aug.; 18(4): 303–7.

16. Barber, A. E. "Glutamine or fiber supplementation of a defined formula diet: impact on bacterial translocation, tissue composition, and response to endotoxin." *JPEN.* 1990 July–Aug.; 14(4): 335–43.

17. Slotwinski, R. "Cellular immunity changes after total parenteral nutrition enriched with glutamine in patients with sepsis and malnutrition." *Pol Merkur Lekarski.* 2000 June; 8(48): 405–408.

18. Bamba, T. "A new prebiotic from germinated barley for nutraceutical treatment of ulcerative colitis." *J Gastroenterol Hepatol.* 2002 Aug.; 17(8): 818–24.

19. Zhang, W. "Glutamine reduces bacterial translocation after small bowel transplantation in cyclosporine-treated rats." *J Surg Res.* 1995 Feb.; 58(2): 159–64.

20. Rosenbloom, C. "Contemporary ergogenic aids used by strength/power athletes." *JADA.* 1992 Oct.; 92(10): 1264–66.

21. Accinni, R. "Effects of combined dietary supplementation on oxidative and inflammatory status in dyslipidemic subjects." *Nutr Metb Cardiovasc. Dis* 2006 March; 16(2): 121–27.

22. Sierra, S. "Increased immune response in mice consuming rice bran oil." *Eur Jrnl Nutr.* 2005 Dec.; 44(8): 509–16.

23. Jariwalla, R. J. "Rice-bran products: phytonutrients with potential applications in preventive and clinical medicine." *Drugs Exp Clin Res.* 2001; 27(1): 17–26.

24. Xu, Z. "Antioxidant activity of tocopherols, tocotrienols, and gamma–oryzanol components from rice bran against cholesterol oxidation accelerated by 2,2'-azobis(2-methylpropionamidine) dihydrochloride." *Jrnl Agric Food Chem.* 2001 April; 49(4): 2077–81.

Chapter 10

1. *FDA Consumer.* "Can Your Kitchen Pass the Food Safety Test?" revised July 2002 (http://www.cfsan.fda.gov/~dms/fdkitchn.html).

2. *FDA Consumer.* "The Unwelcome Dinner Guest Preventing Food-Borne Illness." Revised March 2003 (http://www.fda.gov/fdac/reprints/dinguest.html).

3. Hertzler, S. R. "Improved lactose digestion and intolerance among African-American adolescent girls fed a dairy-rich diet." *Am Diet Assoc.* 2000 May; 100(5): 524–28.

4. Kevers, C. "Evolution of antioxidant capacity during storage of selected fruits and vegetables." *J Agric Food Chem.* 2007 Oct. 17; 55(21): 8596.

5. Kosa, K. M. "Consumer home refrigeration practices: results of a web-based survey." *J Food Prot.* 2007 July; 70(7): 1640–49.

6. Blake, T. K. "Journaling; an active learning technique." *Int J Nurs Educ Scholarsh.* 2005; 2: Article 7.

7. Burke, L. E. "Using instrumented paper diaries to document self-monitoring patterns in weight loss." *Contemp Clin.* 2007 July 25.

Chapter 11

1. Tuohy, K. M. "Using Probiotics and Prebiotics to Improve Gut Health." *Drug Disc Today.* 2003 Aug. 1; 8(15): 692–700.

2. Campbell, A. P. "Flax, a Grain for Good Health." *Diabetes Self-Manag.* 2003 Nov.–Dec.; 20(6): 18, 20–22.

3. Siddiqui, R. A. "Omega-3 fatty acids: health benefits and cellular mechanisms of action." *Mini Rev Med Chem.* 2004 Oct.; 4(8): 859–71.

Chapter 12

1. Mayo Clinic. "Health tips. Sources of soluble fiber." *Mayo Clin Health Lett.* 2007 Aug.; 25(8):3.
2. McKee, L. H. "Underutilized sources of dietary fiber: a review." *Plant Foods Hum Nutr.* 2000; 55(4): 285–304.
3. Mumy, K. L. "Saccharomyces boulardii interferes with Shigella pathogenesis by post-invasion signaling events." *Am J Physiol Gastrointest Liver Physiol.* 2007 Nov. 21.
4. Talegawkar, S. A. "Carotenoid intakes, assessed by food–frequency question-naires (FFQs), are associated with serum carotenoid concentrations in the Jackson Heart Study: validation of the Jackson Heart Study Delta NIRI Adult FFQs." *Public Health Nutr.* 2007 Dec 6; 1–9.
5. Monagas, M. "Almond (Prunus dulcis [Mill.] D.A. Webb) skins as a potential source of bioactive polyphenols." *J Agric Food Chem.* 2007 Oct. 17; 55(21): 8498–8507.
6. Gorinstein, S. "The atherosclerotic heart disease and protecting properties of garlic: contemporary data." *Mol Nutr Food Res.* 2007 Nov.; 51(11): 1365–81.
7. Lee, I. O. "Anti–inflammatory effect of capsaicin in Helicobacter pylori–infected gastric epithelial cells." *Helicobacter.* 2007 Oct.; 12(5): 510–17.
8. Berti, C. "Effect on appetite control of minor cereal and pseudocereal products." *Brit J Nutr.* 2005 Nov.; 94(5): 850–58.
9. Ding, H. "Chemopreventive characteristics of avocado fruit." *Semin Cancer Biol.* 2007 Oct.; 17(5): 386–94.
10. Kleesen, B. "Jerusalem artichoke and chicory inulin in bakery products affect faecal microbiota of healthy volunteers." *Brit J Nutr.* 2007 Sept.; 98(3): 540–49.
11. Lichtenthaler, R. "Total oxidant scavenging capacities of common European fruit and vegetable juices." *J Agric Food Chem.* 2005 Jan. 12: 53.
12. Huang, Z. "Total phenolics and antioxidant capacity of indigenous vegetables in the southeast United States: Alabama Collaboration for Cardiovascular Equality Project." *Int J Food Sci Nutr.* 2007 Sept. 18: 1–9.
13. Hu, C. "Antioxidant activities of the flaxseed lignan secoisolariciresinol digluco-side, its aglycone secoisolariciresinol and the mammalian lignans enterodiol and enterolactone in vitro." *Food Chem Toxicol.* 2007 Nov.; 45(11): 2219–27.

Chapter 13

1. Boynton, A. "Associations between healthy eating patterns and immune function or inflammation in overweight or obese postmenopausal women." *Am J Clin Nutr.* 2007 Nov.; 86(5): 1445–55.
2. Bullo, M. "Inflammation, obesity and comorbidities: the role of diet." *Public Health Nutr.* 2007 Oct.; 10(10A): 1164–72.

3. Jimenez Escrig, A. "Multifunctional in vitro antioxidant evaluation of strawberry (Fragaria virginiana Dutch)." *Int J Food Sci Nutr.* 2007 June 5: 1–8.

4. Yuan, Y. V. "Antioxidant and antiproliferative activities of extracts from a variety of edible seaweeds." *Food Chem Toxicol.* 2006 July; 44(7): 1144–50.

5. Herrera, I. M. "Soluble, insoluble and total dietary fiber in raw and cooked legumes." *Arch Latinoam Nutr.* 1998 June; 48(2): 179–82.

6. Kamei, H. "Suppression of growth of cultured malignant cells by allomelanins, plant-produced melanins." *Cancer Biother Radiopharm.* 1997 Feb.; 12(1): 47–49.

7. Ogbolu, D. O. "In vitro antimicrobial properties of coconut oil on Candida species in Ibadan, Nigeria." *J Med Food.* 2007 June; 10(2): 384–87.

Chapter 14

1. Simcox, N. J. "Pesticides in household dust and soil." *Environ Health Persp.* 1995 Dec.; 103(12): 1126–34.

2. Hunt, A. "Mass transfer of soil indoors by track-in on footwear." *Sci Total Environ.* 2006 Nov. 1; 370(2–3): 360–71.

3. Redmond, E. C. "Consumer Food Handling in the Home: a review of food safety studies." *J Food Protect.* 2003 Jan.; 66(1): 130–61.

4. *Food Safety Fact Sheet.* Illinois Department of Public Health, 525 W. Jefferson St., Springfield, IL 62761 (http://www.idph.state.il.us/about/fdd/fdd_fs_foodservice.htm).

5. *Safe Food Handling Fact Sheets.* USDA, Food Safety and Inspection Service, www.fsis.usda.gov/Fact_Sheets/Safe_Food_Handling_Fact_Sheets/index.asp

6. Harada, K. "Case study of volatile organic compounds in indoor air of a house before and after repair where sick building syndrome occurred." *Int J Immunopathol Pharmacol.* 2007 April–June; 20(2 Suppl 2): 69–74.

7. Nakayama, K. "Relationship between lifestyle, mold and sick building syndromes in newly built dwellings in Japan." *Int J Immunopathol Pharmacol.* 2007 April–June; 20(2 Suppl 2): 35–43.

8. Hope, A. P. "Excess dampness and mold growth in homes." *Allergy Asthma Proc.* 2007 May–June; 28(3): 262–70.

9. Zhang, Z. "Variation in yearly residential radon concentrations in the upper midwest." *Health Phys.* 2007 Oct.; 93(4): 288–97.

10. Sharmer, L. "Newly recognized pathways of exposure to lead in the middle-income home." *J Environ Health.* 2007 Oct.; 70(3): 15–19, 48.

11. Gorfine, T. "Late evening brain activation patterns and their relation to the internal biological time, melatonin, and homeostatic sleep debt." *Hum Brain Mapp.* 2007 Dec. 19.

12. Staskel, D. M. "Microbial evaluation of food-service surfaces in Texas child-care centers." *J Am Diet Assoc.* 2007 May; 107(5): 854–59.

13. Singer, B. C. "Cleaning products and air fresheners: emissions and resulting concentrations of glycol ethers and terpenoids." *Indoor Air.* 2006 June; 16(3): 179–91.

14. Campanha, N. H. "Candida albicans inactivation and cell membrane integrity damage by microwave irradiation." *Mycoses.* 2007 March; 50(2): 140–47.

15. Thompson, R. C. "The public health and clinical significance of Giardia and Cryptosporidium in domestic animals." *Vet J.* 2007 Nov. 19.

16. Beazley, D. M. "Toxoplasmosis." *Semin Perinatol.* 1998 Aug.; 22(4): 332–38.

17. Nedorost, S. "Allergens retained in clothing." *Dermatitis.* 2007 Dec.; 18(4): 212–14.

18. Rocha-Amador, "Decreased intelligence in children and exposure to fluoride and arsenic in drinking water." *Cad Saude Publica.* 2007; 23 (Suppl 4): S579–87.

19. Masanova, V. "Manganese and copper imbalance in the food chain constituents in relation to Creutzfeldt–Jakob disease." *Int J Environ Health Res.* 2007 Dec.; 17(6): 419–28.

20. Saber-Tehrani, M. "Assessment of some elements in human permanent healthy teeth, their dependence on number of metallic amalgam fillings, and interelements relationships." *Biol Trace Elem Res.* 2007 May; 116(2): 155–69.

Chapter 15

1. Reilly, T. "Nutrition for travel." *J Sports Sci.* 2007 Dec.; 25 (Suppl 1): 125–34.

2. McMullan, R. "Food-poisoning and commercial air travel." *Travel Med Infect Dis.* 2007 Sept.; 5(5): 276–86.

3. DeHart, R. L. "Health Issues of Air Travel," *Annu Rev of Public Hlth.* 2003; 24: 133–51.

4. Caumes, E. "Common diseases after travel in tropical countries." *Rev Prat.* 2007 April 30; 57(8): 845–51.

5. Juneja, V. K. "A comparative heat inactivation study of indigenous microflora in beef with that of Listeria monocytogenes, Salmonella serotypes and Escherichia coli O157:H7. *Lett Appl Microbiol.* 2003; 37(4): 292–98.

6. Sanford, C. "Pre-travel advice: an overview." *Prim Care.* 2002 Dec.; 29(4): 767–85.

7. Lee, C. C. "Foodborne diseases." *Singapore Med J.* 1996 April; 37(2): 197–204.

8. Oussalah, M. "Mechanism of action of Spanish oregano, Chinese cinnamon, and savory essential oils against cell membranes and walls of Escherichia coli O157:H7 and Listeria monocytogenes. *J Food Prot.* 2006 May; 69(5): 1046–55.

9. Paez Jimenez, A. "Waterborne outbreak among Spanish tourists in a holiday resort in the Dominican Republic, August 2002." *Euro Surveil.* 2004 March; 9(3) 21–23.

10. Schlosser, O. "Bacterial removal from inexpensive portable water treatment systems for traveler." *J Travel Med.* 2001 Jan.–Feb.; 8(1): 12–8.

11. Backer, H. "Use of iodine for water disinfection: iodine toxicity and maximum recommended dose." *Environ Health Persp.* 2000 Aug.; 108(8): 679–84.

12. Cohen, P. R. "Community-acquired methicillin-resistant Staphylococcus aureus: skin infection presenting as an axillary abscess with cellulitis in a college athlete." *Skinmed.* 2005 March–April; 4(2): 115–18.

13. Arnold, F. W. "An analysis of a community-acquired pathogen in a Kentucky community: methicillin-resistant Staphylococcus aureus." *J Ky Med Assoc.* 2005 May; 103(5): 206–10.

14. Oie, S. "Association between Isolation Sites of Methicillin-Resistant Staphylococcus aureus (MRSA) in Patients with MRSA-Positive Body Sites and MRSA Contaminaton in Their Surrounding Environmental Surfaces." *Japanese J Infect Dis.* 2007 Nov.; 60(6): 367–69.

15. Edge, T. A. "Experience with the antibiotic resistance analysis and DNA fingerprinting in tracking faecal pollution at two lake beaches." *Water Sci Technol.* 2007; 56(11): 51–58.

16. Ritter, L. "Sources, pathways, and relative risks of contaminants in surface water and groundwater: a perspective prepared for the Walkerton inquiry." *J Toxicol Environ Health A.* 2002 Jan. 11; 65(1): 1–142.

17. Benedict, M. Q. "Spread of the tiger: global risk of invasion by the mosquito Aedes albopictus." *Vector Borne Zoonotic Dis.* 2007 Spring; 7(1): 76–85.

18. Fradin, M. S. "Comparitive efficacy of insect repellents against mosquito bites." *NEJM* 2002, July 4; 347(1): 13–18.

19. Ordinioha, B. "The use of insecticide-treated bed net in a semi-urban community in south-south, Nigeria." *Niger J Med.* 2007 July–Sept.; 16(3): 223–36.

20. Adams, H.S. "Fine particle (PM2.5) personal exposure levels in transport microenvironments, London, UK." *Sci Total Environ.* 2001 Nov. 12; 279(1–3): 29–44.

21. McNabola, A. "Reduced exposure to air pollution on the boardwalk in Dublin, Ireland. Measurement and prediction." *Environ Int.* 2008 Jan.; 34(1): 86–89.

22. Baumann, L.S. "Less-known botanical cosmeceuticals." *Dermatol Ther.* 2007 Sept.–Oct.; 20(5) 330–42.

23. Spiel, C. "Fever of unknown origin in the returning traveler." *Infect Dis Clin North Am.* 2007 Dec.; 21(4): 1091–1113.

Chapter 16

1. Rogers, P. M. "Human adenovirus Ad-36 induces adipogenesis via its E4 orf-1 gene." *Int J Obes* (Lond). 2007 Nov. 6.

2. Atkinson, R. L. "Viruses as an etiology of obesity." *Mayo Clin Proc.* 2007 Oct.; 82(10): 1192–98.

3. Bern, C. "Evaluation and treatment of Chagas' disease in the United States: a systematic review." *JAMA*, 2007 Nov. 14; 298(18): 2171–81.

4. Karanis, P. "Waterborne transmission of protozoan parasites: a worldwide review of outbreaks and lessons learnt." *J Water Health*. 2007 March; 5(1): 1–38.

5. Grate, I., Jr. "Primary amebic meningoencephalitis: a silent killer." *CJEM*. 2006 Sept.; 8(5): 365–69.

6. Awadzi, K. "The effects of high-dose ivermectin regimens on Onchocerca volvulus in onchocerciasis patients." *Trans R Soc Trop Med Hyg*. 1999 March–April; 93(2): 189–94.

7. Stasinakis, A. S. "Occurrence and fate of endocrine disrupters in Greek sewage treatment plants." *Water Res*. 2007 Nov. 17.

8. Godwin, C. "Indoor air quality in Michigan schools." *Indoor Air*. 2007 April; 17(2): 109–21.

9. Rumchev, K. "Volatile organic compounds: do they present a risk to our health?" *Rev Environ Health*. 2007 Jan.–March; 22(1): 39–5.

10. Caress, S. M. "A national population study of the prevalence of multiple chemical sensitivity." *Arch Environ Health*. 2004 June; 59(6): 300–305.

11. Aarstrup, F. M. "Comparison of antimicrobial resistance phenotypes and resistance genes in Enterococcus faecalis and Enterococcus faecium from humans in the community, broilers, and pigs in Denmark." *Diagn Microbiol Infect Dis*. 2000 June; 37(2): 127–37.

12. "FDA withdraws approval of two poultry drugs." *FDA Consumer*. 2001 July–Aug.; 35(4): 5.

13. Leser, T. D. "Germination and outgrowth of Bacillus subtilis and Bacillus licheniformis spores in the gastrointestinal tracts of pigs." *J Appl Microbiol*. 2007 Nov. 15.

14. Quigley, E. M. "Bacteria: a new player in gastrointestinal motility disorders—infections, bacterial overgrowth, and probiotics." *Gastroenterol Clin North Am*. 2007 Sept.; 36(3): 735–48, xi.

15. Senchina, D. S. "Immunological outcomes of exercise in older adults." *Clin Interv Aging*. 2007; 2(1): 3–16.

16. Pettee, K. K. "Influence of marital status on physical activity levels among older adults." *Med Sci Sports Exerc*. 2006 March; 38(3): 541–46.

17. Wallace, J. P. "Twelve-month adherence of adults who joined a fitness program with a spouse vs. without a spouse." *J Sports Med Phys Fitness*. 1995 Sept.; 35(3): 206–13.

Resources

Gut Flush Supplements and Other Recommended Resources

Uni Key Health Systems
181 West Commerce Drive
Hayden Lake, ID 83838
800-888-4353
unikey@unikeyhealth.com
www.unikeyhealth.com

As the official distributor of all my products and books, Uni Key carries:

- Dr. Ohhira's Probiotics 12 PLUS
- Super-GI Cleanse
- HCl + 2
- Carlson's fish oil and softgels
- Flaxseed oil and softgels
- My Colon Cleansing Kit, which includes a thirty-day supply of Para-Key, Verma-Plus, and Flora-Key (also can be purchased separately)
- Y-C Cleanse
- Thorne SF722

- Zymex II
- Thorne Sacro-B (Saccharomyces boulardii)
- Carlson's L-glutamine powder
- American Biologics Ultra Inf-Zyme Forte
- Standard Process Cholacol
- Doulton water filters
- Dandelion root tea bags and capsules
- Fat Flush Whey, one of the only commercially available unheated, undenatured whey protein concentrate protein powders made from milk that is hormone-free
- Dr. Ohhira's probiotic soap, a much safer alternative to the antibacterial cleansers that are on the market

Uni Key can provide you with a do-it-yourself stool sample kit to help identify parasite and yeast infestations. Your sample is sent to the Parasitology Center in Tempe, Arizona, where it is examined for more than a dozen protozoa, fifteen types of worms, all the common yeasts (including Candida albicans), and fungi spores. A personal letter with recommendations is then sent back to you from my office.

Another do-it-yourself test helpful in fighting yeast is the tissue mineral analysis, which Uni Key offers. This analysis includes a full report, up to twenty pages, which graphically illustrates the levels of thirty-two major minerals (including yeast-related copper) and six toxic metals in the body. Each mineral is fully evaluated in terms of its relationship with other minerals. There is also a complete discussion of your disease tendencies based on mineral levels and ratios.

Gut Flush Forum

www.annlouise.com/forum

Visit my Web site for the Gut Flush Forum created specially for the readers of this book. My moderators and online community are waiting to assist you 24/7. They will gladly answer your questions from this book and offer support as you travel down the amazing path toward gut wellness. You can also connect with other Gut Flushers and swap experiences, tips, and tricks about how to follow the plan. A special feature of the forum is a tantalizing recipe collection that coordinates with the Gut Flush Plan.

Custom Nutritional and Medical Services

Personal Meal Planning Services

Linda Shapiro
Naples, Florida
Linda@personalmealplanning.com

These days, maintaining a healthy eating lifestyle takes commitment as we struggle to balance our time between work, family, and personal obligations. Linda Shapiro, the recipe moderator on www.annlouise.com/forum, can help by providing personalized meal analysis and meal-planning services for all of my programs, including the Gut Flush Plan.

Personalized Medical Consultation

(If you decide to use medications under a doctor's supervision, please make sure you test your stool regularly at least every other month to monitor progress and also test your blood to assess liver enzymes, as medication can be hard on a sensitized system.)

Shirley B. Scott, M.D., P.C.
P.O. Box 2670
Santa Fe, NM 87504
505-986-9960

In many cases, natural remedies relieve gut-related issues. But when stronger measures are needed, Shirley B. Scott, M.D., excels. Many years ago, I worked with Dr. Scott and shared my research and passion for parasites. Dr. Scott has since taken up the medical mantle and is the only doctor in the country that I can recommend for individualized consultation when your condition is more complex. Dr. Scott is extraordinarily knowledgeable about the most accurate lab testing and how to get rid of infectious organisms that require medication and medical follow-through.

Personalized Dental Consultation

Hal H. Huggins, DDS, M.S.
5082 List Drive
Colorado Springs, CO 80919
866-948-4638
Fax: 719-548-8229
email@hugnet.com
www.DrHuggins.com

Dr. Huggins is a pioneer in correcting imbalances in body chemistry caused by dental materials or dental procedures. He believes that many incurable or unresolved diseases involving the immune system, GI tract, heart, lungs, and overall health can be linked to incompatible dental materials, bridges, crowns, root canals, impacted wisdom teeth, and cavitations (as in my personal case). He offers an Alliance of associated dentists throughout the country who follow his specific protocols and many books and videos regarding his cutting-edge work.

Testing

Testing Your Doctor Can Order

Diagnos-Techs, Inc.
6620 South 192nd Place, Building J
Kent, WA 98032
800-878-3787
Fax: 425-251-0637
Diagnos@diagnostechs.com
http://www.diagnostechs.com/

Diagnos-Techs, established in 1987, offers the GI Health Panel™, a noninvasive screen of the gastrointestinal tract and its function that includes fifteen to twenty-two individual but related tests. In these tests, you collect stool and saliva samples at home and then submit them. The lab performs stool antigen and saliva antibody tests like the biochemical E. histolytica saliva antibody that can distinguish between pathogenic and nonpathogenic types of amoeba. Diagnos-Techs employs a variety of methods in the GI Health Panel tests that are highly effective in detecting and identifying pathogens and that use proven biochemical and state-of-the-art immunological methods.

The GI Health Panel includes: 1) pathogen screening for bacteria, fungi, yeast, and various parasites; and 2) digestion-related screening to determine enzyme levels and immunochemical markers for intolerance to common offending foods. Intestinal function markers are used to evaluate irritation and inflammation. These markers, such as occult blood, indicate overall status of gut immunity and integrity. (You need a doctor's referral for this test.)

Metametrix Clinical Laboratory
3425 Corporate Way
Duluth, GA 30096
800-221-4640
Fax: 770-441-2237
www.metametrix.com
inquiries@metametrix.com

Metametrix Clinical Laboratory specializes in measuring nutritional, metabolic, and toxic influences on health. Metametrix offers the GI Effects Stool Profiles, which employs DNA analysis to identify microbiota (including anaerobes) with high accuracy. In addition to comprehensive bacteriology, mycology, and parasitology, GI Effects Stool Profiles recognizes drug-resistant genes, antibiotic and botanical sensitivities, gliadin-specific sIgA, Elastase, plus other inflammation, digestion, and absorption markers. Call to obtain a doctor's referral in your area.

Jetti Katz Tropical Medicine Laboratory
800-A Fifth Avenue, Suite 203
New York, NY 10021
212-207-4923
Fax: 212-207-4920
http://www.jettikatzlab.com

The Jetti Katz Tropical Medicine Laboratory, established eighty years ago, performs stool testing for intestinal parasites, bacteria, and toxins.

Water Filter Testing
NSF International
789 North Dixboro Road

P.O. Box 130140
Ann Arbor, MI 48113-0140
877-867-3435
Fax: 313-769-0109
http://www.NSF.org/certified/DWTU/

For more information about water filters, contact NSF International, an independent testing company that performs tests on filters and certifies them according to how well they remove protozoan parasites. The organization does not, however, measure how effective filters are against viruses and bacteria.

Food Sensitivities and Allergy Testing

EnteroLab
Specialized Laboratory Testing for Optimal Intestinal and Overall Health
10875 Plano Road
Suite 123
Dallas, TX 75238
972-686-6869
www.enterolab.com

EnteroLab is an accredited clinical laboratory specializing in the analysis of intestinal specimens for immune reactions to gluten (contained in wheat, barley, rye, and oats) and other sensitivities to common dietary proteins, which are often the root causes of chronic health problems.

EnteroLab has its own particular screening test for immune sensitivity to gluten, dietary yeast (Saccharomyces cerevisiae), cow's milk, egg, soy, and other foods. Their test examines stool to detect immunological reactions to dietary proteins within the intestinal tract. Recent research at EnteroLab.com indicates that up to four of ten Americans suffer an immune sensitivity to gluten.

Immuno Laboratories, Inc.
6801 Powerline Road
Fort Lauderdale, FL 33309
954-691-2500
800-231-9197
Fax: 954-691-2505
www.immunolabs.com

Established in 1978, Immuno Laboratories provides personalized testing that is available via a personal physician or through a physician referral service. Along with offering support from their nutritionists, they offer a ninety-day guarantee on their services.

Sage Medical Laboratory
Delayed Food Allergy Testing and Treatment for the Relief of Chronic
  Illnesses
1400 Hand Avenue, Suite L
Ormond Beach, FL 32174
877-724-3522
Fax: 386-615-2027
www.foodallergytest.com

Sage was established by Brent Dorval, Ph.D., an MIT visiting scholar and laboratory immunologist, and Daniel C. Dantini, M.D., a practicing physician. It specializes in testing for delayed food allergies, which can be related to gastrointestinal, neurological conditions, lung, chest, dermatologic, ear, nose, and throat, musculoskeletal, genitourinary, cardiovascular, and endocrine problems.

Overall Health Testing
Your Future Health
P.O. Box 1369
Tavares, FL 32778
877-468-6934
www.yourfuturehealth.com

Your Future Health specializes in customized testing for blood, stool, and urine and nutritionally oriented interpretations. YFH offers the services of house visits by phlebotomists to draw your blood at home.

The company also makes available complete testing kits that include the shipping and tracking fees for overnight delivery of samples back to the lab for analysis, the blood draw fees for licensed phlebotomists, the lab analysis fees for the lab best suited to perform your tests, and an interpretation based on their thirty-year database of proprietary statistical data. Their results are transmitted directly from the lab via YFH's customized computer programming.

As many of my readers and followers know, I personally test with YFH regularly and have for years because of their attention to detail, as well as their customer-friendly testing system. With the evidence they provide, I can quickly identify what nutritional levels need adjustment in time to detect an imbalance at the very earliest stage before patterns become manifest on the physical level. For many of my clients, this has been lifesaving.

Associations

International Association for Colon Hydrotherapy
P.O. Box 461285
San Antonio, TX 78246-1285
210-366-2888
Fax: 210-366-2999
www.i-act.org

Colon hydrotherapists flush out wastes from the large intestine with filtered and temperature-regulated water. The water softens and loosens the colon's contents, which is then evacuated through natural peristalsis. Colon hydrotherapy works best when combined with adequate nutrient and fluid intake and exercise. Modern improvements to hydrotherapy's sophisticated technology has made this treatment safe and sanitary.

The International Association for Colon Hydrotherapy (I-ACT)

- certifies and recertifies colon hydrotherapy practitioners;
- maintains a set of competency standards for safety;
- promotes uniform standards of practice and ethical conduct;
- offers referrals to practitioners.

Healing Waters Colon Hydrotherapy
810 Mandeville Lane, Suite 2A
Bozeman, MT 59715
406-586-5515

Healing Waters is very familiar with the Gut Flush protocols and products. I highly recommend Certified Colon Hydrotherapist Georgia Cold's services.

LifeLink Association
411 South 13th Street
Coeur D'Alene, ID 83814
208-765-3082
joankmoe@yahoo.com

J. Kathie Moe, Certified Colon Hydrotherapist, is my personal colon hydrotherapist, and she has more than twenty years of experience. She is also very familiar with the Gut Flush protocols and products.

Organic Trade Association
P.O. Box 547
Greenfield, MA 01302
413-774-7511
Fax: 413-774-6432
info@ota.com
www.ota.com

The Organic Trade Association (OTA) is the membership-based business association for the organic industry in North America. OTA's mission is to promote and protect organic trade to benefit the environment, farmers, the public, and the economy. OTA envisions organic products becoming a significant part of everyday life, enhancing people's lives and the environment.

OTA represents businesses across the organic supply chain and addresses all things organic, including food, fiber/textiles, personal care products, and new sectors as they develop. More than 60 percent of OTA trade members are small businesses.

VillageOrganics
www.villageorganics.com/organicmarket.html
info@villageorganics.com

VillageOrganics is a family-run online shopping guide to natural and organic foods. All items are sold and shipped by the merchants represented on the site. A portion of the revenues generated by sales are used for humanitarian efforts. All of the food and beverage products offered are USDA Organic or contain certified organic ingredients, are vegetarian according to their listed ingredients, and contain no hydrogenated oils.

LocalHarvest
Community Supported Agriculture
220 21st Avenue
Santa Cruz, CA 95062
831-475-8150
Fax: 831-401-2418
www.LocalHarvest.org/csa

LocalHarvest, a Web site featuring organic and locally grown foods, maintains a public nationwide "living" directory of small farms, farmers' markets, and other local food sources. Its search engine helps people find products from family farms and local sources of sustainably grown food, and encourages direct contact with small farms in their local area. The online store helps small farms develop markets for some of their products beyond their local areas. Many farms in its database offer produce subscriptions, allowing you to receive a weekly or monthly basket of produce, flowers, fruits, eggs, or other farm products.

Nutrition Education

Clayton College of Natural Health
2140 11th Avenue South, Suite 305
Birmingham, AL 35205
800-659-2426
205-323-8246
communications@ccnh.edu
www.ccnh.edu

Clayton College offers college degree programs in natural health and holistic nutrition through distance education. These programs provide students with a wide variety of tools with which they can educate others in achieving and maintaining health through the use of natural elements such as proper diet, pure water, clean air, exercise, and rest. In addition to degree programs in natural health and holistic nutrition, CCNH offers certificate and/or concentration programs in herbal studies, nutrition and lifestyles, and iridology.

American College of Nutrition
300 South Duncan Avenue, Suite 225
Clearwater, FL 33755

727-446-6086 or 727-446-7958
Fax: 727-446-6202
office@am-coll-nutr.org

The American College of Nutrition was established in 1959 to promote scientific endeavors in the field of nutritional sciences.

The National Institute of Whole Health

The New England School of Whole Health Education
3 Cameron Place
Wellesley, MA 02482
888-354-HEAL (4325)
Fax: 781-431-0017
info@wholehealtheducation.org
www.wholehealtheducation.com

Established in 1977, NIWH offers comprehensive Whole Health certification programs. The organization's holistic health education DVD courses utilize evidence-based curriculums to integrate holistic health care concepts, natural health science, and whole person health care training in a distance learning format.

Professionally Accredited Whole Health Certifications for Qualified Students allow you to earn credentials to work in health care jobs such as nutrition educator, health educator, and health coaching, with professionally accredited, evidence-based certifications from the most trusted Whole Health program in the country.

Certification Board for Nutrition Specialists

Att: Pearl Small, CBNS Coordinator
300 South Duncan Avenue, Suite 225
Clearwater, FL 33755
727-446-6086, ext 103
Fax: 727-446-6202
office@cbns.org
www.cbns.org

Founded in 1993 by the American College of Nutrition, the Certification Board for Nutrition Specialists was created as a national certifying body for the advanced degree of nutritionist (master's and doctoral level) from regionally accredited institutions that desired more formal recognition of their skills, knowledge, and experience. CBNS certification allows the public a way to distinguish highly trained, competent nutritionists with confidence and assurance. The protected title of Certified Nutrition Specialist (CNS) is awarded by CBNS to those nutritionists meeting defined educational, experience, and examination requirements. Continuing education requirements help ensure that standards of excellence are maintained. CNS diplomats are found in a variety of professional settings in private practice, public and community health care, universities, and industry. Since 1998, CBNS certification has been extended to include physicians with similar expertise and experience in basic and applied nutrition. Some of the most recognized names in the field of nutrition hold the CNS credential.

Celiac Resources

Celiac Disease and Gluten-free Diet Support Center

www.celiac.com

Celiac Disease and Gluten-free Diet Support Center provides important resources and information for people following gluten-free diets who have celiac disease, gluten intolerance, dermatitis herpetiformis, wheat allergy, and other health issues.

The Celiac Disease Foundation

www.celiac.org

CDF provides support, information, and assistance to people affected by celiac disease/dermatitis herpetiformis (CD/DH). CDF works closely with health care professionals, pharmaceutical, and medical industries. This cooperative effort puts CDF at the forefront of CD/DH care and research, helping to aid and benefit those affected.

The University of Maryland Center for Celiac Research

20 Penn Street, Room S303B
Baltimore, MD 21201
800-492-5538
www.celiaccenter.org

The University of Maryland Center for Celiac Research is dedicated to improving the quality of life for celiac patients while researching the cause of the disease and finding a cure. Located in downtown Baltimore, the Center for Celiac Research provides comprehensive clinical care and long-term support for adults and children who suffer from this genetically based autoimmune disease, which the center believes affects 1 out of every 133 people in the United States.

glutenfree.com
P.O. Box 840
Glastonbury, CT 06033
800-291-8386

Since 1995, Celiac Disease Diet Food Products (glutenfree.com) has been offering organic gluten-free products to people with gluten sensitivities. The company was founded by professional chef and food writer Beth Hillson, who, along with her son, follows a gluten-free diet.

Gluten-Free Restaurant Awareness Program
feedback@glutenfreerestaurants.org
www.glutenfreerestaurants.org

The Gluten-Free Restaurant Awareness Program (GFRAP) was formed to make it easier to stay on a gluten-free diet while dining out. It helps restaurants create products for people on gluten-free diets, helps consumers find suitable restaurants, and educates participating restaurants in ways to provide gluten-free meals along with conventional dishes. GFRAP is a program of the Gluten Intolerance Group of North America.

Karina's Kitchen
glutenfreegoddess.blogspot.com

This blog features more than two hundred original recipes from Karina Allrich's kitchen. Her mantra: "Life is short—make today delicious."

Recommended Books, Magazines, Newsletters, and Web Sites
Books
Guess What Came to Dinner? Parasites and Your Health
(Revised and Updated)

Ann Louise Gittleman, Ph.D., CNS

Avery, second edition, 2001

This is the "underground classic" that was years ahead of its time and opened a real can of worms. Thanks to the pioneering research in this book, many individuals now understand that parasites are alive and well in twenty-first-century America and that they can learn how to protect themselves and their families from an alarming epidemic that knows no economic or social boundaries. Parasites can masquerade as numerous illnesses (irritable bowel syndrome, asthma, obesity, chronic fatigue, insomnia, skin conditions, allergies—even cancer), and this book offers all you need to know and more about parasite warning signs, the water and food connection, threats to and from pets, diagnosis, treatment, and prevention. This book features a unique protocol of natural herbal-based and botanical remedies and enzymes that treat both microscopic parasites and worms in every developmental cycle throughout the body.

The Fat Flush Plan

Ann Louise Gittleman, Ph.D., CNS

McGraw-Hill, 2002

The Fat Flush Plan provides a stringent and regimented three-phase program that can be used in conjunction with the Gut Flush Plan. This book is ideal for individuals that need everything laid out on a daily basis in terms of timing and menus for breakfast, lunch, dinner, and snacks.

The Fat Flush Cookbook

Ann Louise Gittleman, Ph.D., CNS

McGraw-Hill, 2002

The Fat Flush Cookbook provides more than two hundred recipes for breakfasts, snacks, lunches, dinners, desserts, and beverages that are compatible with the Gut Flush Plan.

Breaking the Vicious Cycle: Intestinal Health Through Diet

Elaine Gloria Gottschall

Kirkton Press, revised edition, 1994

In writing *Breaking the Vicious Cycle,* Elaine Gottschall shared what she had learned in the three decades since her four-year-old daughter was diagnosed as having severe, incurable ulcerative colitis. The book documents her uncharted odyssey to keep her child alive and stave off an ileostomy (surgical removal of the colon and replacement with an external bag). A biochemist–cell biologist, Gottschall is convinced that proper nutrition is often an alternative to heavy medication and surgery and that many diseases can be prevented, alleviated, or cured by nothing more than the correct diet.

Digestive Wellness
Elizabeth Lipski, Ph.D.
McGraw-Hill, 2004

Between 60 and 70 million people suffer from digestive problems according to the National Digestive Diseases Information Clearinghouse. Besides the common cold, digestive problems are the most common reason people seek medical advice. This comprehensive work offers many practical ideas for digestive problems. Lipski brings together all the latest clinical studies on digestion. By throwing the spotlight on this critical function, she shows how far-reaching and essential healthy digestion is to everyone's well-being.

Digestive Wellness for Children: How to Strengthen the Immune System & Prevent Disease Through Healthy Digestion
Elizabeth Lipski, Ph.D.
Basic Health Publications, 2006

Digestive Wellness for Children is a dependable guide to help you improve your children's health by improving their digestion. Not only is faulty digestion directly responsible for a disturbingly large number of gastrointestinal disorders, but it can also be indirectly responsible for a vast array of seemingly unrelated illnesses, including arthritis, migraines, and autoimmune diseases.

No More Heartburn: Stop the Pain in 30 Days—Naturally! The Safe, Effective Way to Prevent and Heal Chronic Gastrointestinal Disorders
Sherry Rodgers, M.D.
Kensington, 2000

Heartburn and indigestion are common ailments that are all too often, and wrongly, treated by prescription and over-the-counter drugs that mask the symptoms and ignore the underlying, often serious, causes. In this book, Dr. Sherry Rogers, a leading expert in drug-free gastrointestinal therapy, explains how to pinpoint the causes of your stomach distress and offers easy-to-follow advice for creating an effective, personalized program for achieving and maintaining total gastrointestinal health.

Eat Well, Feel Well: More Than 150 Delicious Specific Carbohydrate Diet™ Compliant Recipes
Kendall Conrad
Clarkson Potter, 2006

When her daughter was diagnosed with a dangerous digestive problem that left her weakened and sick, author Kendall Conrad started searching for a way to save her child's failing health. She found the answer when a nutritionist recommended the Specific Carbohydrate Diet (SCD) created by Elaine Gottschall. This revolutionary program is extraordinarily effective in relieving the debilitating and often painful symptoms of ulcerative colitis, celiac disease, diverticulitis, IBS, Crohn's disease, and other common ailments. By simply eliminating virtually all starch and complex sugars and eating a balance of smart carbohydrates, good proteins and fats, as well as essential vitamins and minerals, many people on the SCD experience a complete restoration of digestive health. For Conrad's daughter, the results were lifesaving. This book includes recipes for the whole family that follow Gottschall's guidelines.

The Probiotics Revolution: The Definitive Guide to Safe, Natural Health Solutions Using Probiotic and Prebiotic Foods and Supplements
Gary B. Huffnagle, Ph.D., and Sarah Wernick, Ph.D.
Bantam, 2007

Here is an up-to-the-minute, easy to understand guide to probiotics and the foods and supplements that contain and support them. This book offers insight into the key role probiotics and prebiotics play in restoring healthy balance to our bodies, improving immune system functioning, and curbing inflammation. It also includes advice on using probiotic foods and supplements to prevent and relieve allergies, inflammatory bowel disease, irritable bowel syndrome, and yeast infections. In addition, it discusses the negative side effects of antibiotics.

Going Against the Grain
Melissa Diane Smith
McGraw-Hill/Contemporary Books, 2002

Diets high in grains can lead to a host of health problems such as obesity, diabetes, heart disease, and fatigue. *Going Against the Grain* outlines the disadvantages and potential dangers of eating various types of grains and provides practical, realistic advice on implementing a plan to cut back or eliminate grains on a daily basis.

Magazines

Totalhealth for Longevity magazine
165 North 100 East, Suite #2
St. George, UT 84770-9963
800-788-7806
www.totalhealthmagazine.com

I am fortunate to serve as an associate editor for *Totalhealth for Longevity* magazine. It is a comprehensive voice on antiaging, longevity, and self-managed natural health. Lyle Hurd, publisher extraordinaire, strives to bring readers fresh new information and perspectives on all phases of longevity medicine so that you can make an educated decision on the quality of your life today . . . and tomorrow.

Taste for Life magazine
86 Elm Street
Peterborough, NH 03458
603-924-9692
www.tasteforlife.com

Taste for Life is one of the fastest-growing, in-store magazines for health food stores, natural product chains, food co-ops, and supermarkets nationwide. Its excellent articles on pertinent health issues offer readers an informative educational source on a variety of levels, including physical fitness. I sit on *Taste for Life*'s editorial board.

First for Women magazine
270 Sylvan Avenue
Englewood Cliffs, NJ 07632

800-938-8312

www.firstforwomen.com

First for Women speaks directly to women about their real-life needs, concerns, and interests. You can also read my monthly advice column, "Nutrition Know-How," which has been featured in *First* since 2003.

Newsletters

The Sinatra Health Report

Published by Phillips Health, LLC

7811 Montrose Road

Potomac, MD 20854

800-211-7643

www.drsinatra.com

Stephen Sinatra, M.D., FACN, CNS, is a board-certified cardiologist and certified bioenergetic analyst with more than twenty years of experience in helping patients prevent and reverse heart disease. *The Sinatra Health Report* is published monthly by Phillips Health. Dr. Sinatra, to his credit, is a big proponent of detoxification, and many of his newsletters discuss current research in the environmental medicine arena.

The Woman's Health Letter

P.O. Box 467939

Atlanta, GA 31146-7939

800-728-2288

Nan Kathryn Fuchs, Ph.D., is the editor of *The Woman's Health Letter* and my kind of nutritionist. Her comments regarding health, nutrition, and medicine as they relate to women are right on target.

Nutrition News

4108 Watkins Drive

Riverside, CA 92507

909-784-7500 or 800-784-7550

www.nutritionnews.com

Siri Khalsa is a wonderful veteran journalist who has been in the business of providing health education for more than twenty-five years. Her easy-to-read newsletter covers a wide variety of contemporary and current topics. It is distributed in health food stores throughout the country, but you can also subscribe directly.

Dr. Jonathan V. Wright's *Nutrition & Healing*
Agora South, LLC
819 North Charles Street
Baltimore, MD 21201
410-223-2611

Nutrition & Healing is dedicated to helping you keep yourself and your family healthy by the safest and most effective means possible. Every month it offers information about diet, vitamins, minerals, herbs, natural hormones, natural energies, and other substances and techniques to prevent and heal illness, while prolonging your healthy life span.

The Health Sciences Institute
Healthier News, LLC
819 North Charles Street
Baltimore, MD 21201

As a member of the professional advisory panel, I can verify that this cutting-edge newsletter is devoted to presenting extraordinary products to its members before those items hit the marketplace. It was the first to break the Ultra H-3 story—the extraordinary formula for arthritis, depression, and antiaging. *The Health Sciences Institute* provides private access to hidden cures, powerful discoveries, breakthrough treatments, and advances in modern, underground medicine.

Web Sites

The Intestinal Health Institute
www.intestinalhealth.org

The Intestinal Health Institute is a not-for-profit organization dedicated to improving intestinal and overall health and nutrition through medical research, public service, and education. The institute originated in the research of Kenneth Fine, M.D., who has studied the ill-health effects, particularly intestinal disorders, that result from gluten sensitivity, microscopic colitis, yeast sensitivity, and other causes of intestinal disease and dysfunction. Based on extensive research, the institute believes that at least 50 percent of all Americans suffer reactions of the immune system to common dietary proteins, particularly gluten, found in wheat, barley, rye, and oats. The institute focuses on damage to the intestine (celiac sprue) that can lead to fatigue, depression, abdominal symptoms, malnutrition, infertility in women, osteoporosis, various neurological syndromes, growth failure in children, autoimmune diseases, and a risk of cancer.

Clean Food Resources

www.foodandwaterwatch.org

This site provides information on the latest seafood bans.

www.localharvest.org

This is a consumer-based site, which can help you find locally grown produce.

www.attra.ncat.org/attra-pub/localfood_dir.php

This site helps you locate community-supported farms and agricultural cooperatives.

Kids and the Specific Carbohydrate Diet

www.Pecanbread.com
www.pecanbread.com/new/local1.html

The Specific Carbohydrate Diet (SCD) is an autism diet based on the research into this devastating disorder. SCD attempts to rectify imbalances of gut pathogens (the microorganisms in the gut) that damage the GI tract and impair the brain function of autistic children. According to scientific studies, these harmful microbes survive because they feed and thrive on carbohydrates that are difficult to digest. Consequently, the SCD is meant to eliminate these pathogens' favorite carbohydrates and starve them out.

www.Scdiet.org

The SCD Web Library, founded in 1996, is an edited, purposeful compilation of Listserv communications of thousands of people who are deriving significant results from dietary adjustments.

There are specific carbohydrates that are troublemakers in the digestive system, especially for those people suffering from Crohn's disease, ulcerative colitis, IBS, and celiac. The purpose of the SCD is to eliminate these carbohydrates and facilitate a healthy, natural, controlled remission.

For the Health Care Professional

The DAVE Project (Digital Atlas of Video Education)
dave1.mgh.harvard.edu

The DAVE Project is a collection of teaching tools consisting of a gastrointestinal endoscopy video atlas and medical lectures and presentations. Physicians are encouraged to submit material, for consideration, that provides new entries which can enrich and expand the atlas.

Government Agencies and Watchdog Groups

The U.S. Food and Drug Administration
www.fda.gov

The Food and Drug Administration site provides updates on the latest foods that have been turned back at the border. These updates are detailed in the "refusals" section.

National Organic Program
202-720-3252
www.ams.usda.gov/nop

This is the USDA Web site that offers the official, exhaustive definition of organic. Basically, this site describes in detail the requirement for raising organic food without synthetic pesticides, petroleum or sewage-sludge–based fertilizers, bioengineering, or ionizing radiation. Meat, poultry, eggs, and dairy products that are labeled organic must be derived from animals that are fed 100 percent organic feed without antibiotics or any growth hormones. A USDA inspector ensures that the farms where organic food is produced meet quality standards before products are labeled "organic."

Food Allergy Alerts
www.fda.gov/opacom/7alerts.html

Here is the Web site where the FDA issues recalls, alerts, and updates on tainted and mislabeled food and medication. You can sign up for e-mail alerts on this site.

Generation Green
800-652-0827
www.generationgreen.org
This Web site keeps you informed about the latest government policies that impact food and the environment. Its quarterly newsletter offers updates on the latest regulations and decisions regarding the food supply.

Nutritionally Oriented Medical Organizations

American College for Advancement in Medicine (ACAM)
23121 Verdugo Drive
Suite 204
Laguna Hills, CA 92653
800-532-3688
949-583-7666
www.acam.org
The members of this professional organization are highly skilled in nutrition and various protocols outlined in this book. Contact ACAM to find doctor-members who can perform the Heidelberg test, which measures gastric acidity and the need for HCl.

The American Academy of Environmental Medicine
7701 East Kellogg, Suite 625
Wichita, KS 67207
316-684-5500
Fax: 316-684-5709
www.aaem.com
Like ACAM, the American Academy of Environmental Medicine is a professional organization that includes doctor-members who are nutritionally oriented.

Index

breads, gluten-free (*cont.*)
  Mega-Grain Quick Bread, 232
  pantry staples, 132, 136
broths, 135

C. difficile, 9, 13
cabbage
  juice, 71
  Simple Homemade Sauerkraut, 229–30
caffeinated drinks, 9, 73, 100–101, 102
calcium absorption, 96
CA-MRSA, 64–65
Candida albicans. *See* yeast overgrowth
canned pantry staples, 138–39
capsaicin, 72, 112
carbohydrates
  Antiparasite Protocol, 54
  Fortify step, 91–92
  Flush step, 108
  Feed step, 124–25
  Specific Carbohydrate Diet, 109–10
  sugar and sweeteners, 91, 108
  yeast overgrowth and, 34, 39
  See also beans and legumes
Carrot Soup, Quick and Easy, 240–41
castor oil packs, 103
cayenne, 72, 111–12, 166
celiac disease. *See* gluten sensitivity and celiac
    disease
cereals for pantry staples, 138
Chicken, Amaranth and Herb-Crusted, 237–38
chicory root, 101
Chili with a Twist, Black Bean 'n' Beef, 242
cinnamon, 110–11
climate, yeast overgrowth and, 33
coconut oil, 107–8, 180
coffee, 9, 73, 100–101, 102
coffee enemas, 128
colon cancer, 11
Colon Corruptors. *See* food sensitivities; parasites;
    Superbugs; yeast overgrowth
colonic cleansing, 55, 116–17, 118, 128
community-associated Methicillin-resistant Staphy-
    lococcus aureus, 64–65
condiments for pantry staples, 138
constipation, 7–8
copper, limiting exposure to, 198–99
corn, sensitivity to, 84, 92
crackers for pantry staples, 137–38
Creamy Kabocha Squash Soup, 239–40
Crook, William, 36

dairy products
  Ann Louise's Yogurt, 229
  avoidance of, during travel, 203
  intolerances, 72, 78–80, 84, 134
  pantry staples, 134
dandelion root tea, 101

day-care settings, parasite infestation in, 45
dental cavitations, bacteria in, 30–31
DGL (deglycyrrhizinated licorice), 72–73, 127–28
diagnostic questionnaires and tests
  food sensitivity, 82–83
  HCl stomach acid, 19
  parasites, 51–53
  Superbugs, 68–69
  yeast overgrowth, 36–37
diarrhea, 8–10, 148
digestive enzymes, 25–26, 27
dips and spreads
  Ann Louise's Tangy Tapenade, 233
  Garbanzo Bean Hummus, 233–34
  Parsley and Cilantro Pesto, 234
disruptive digestion, 6
diverticulosis and diverticulitis, 10–11
Dr. Ohhira's Probiotics 12 PLUS, 27, 39, 71,
    94, 96
Dragsted, Lester R., 67
drinks. *See* beverages

E. coli, 21, 63–64, 104
eating programs. *See* menu plans
emotions, 9–10, 142–43
enemas and colonic irrigation, 55, 116–17, 118, 128
environment in home. *See* home environment
enzymes, digestive, 25–26, 27
exercise, 8, 72, 211, 224

fats
  coconut oil, 34, 107–8
  oil of oregano, 40
  olive and sesame oils, 34
  omega-3 fatty acids in fish and flaxseed oils, 34,
    55, 98–99
  pantry staples, 133
Feed step. *See* Week Three
fermented foods
  Ann Louise's Yogurt, 229
  benefits, 93
  enzymes in, 26
  Miso Soup Plus, 230
  Must-Have Miso Dressing, 235
  pantry staples, 134
  sauerkraut, 113, 153
  Simple Homemade Sauerkraut, 229–30
fiber
  in beans, 125
  benefits, 11, 71, 97
  chewing of fibrous foods, 167
  food sources, 71, 97, 98, 125
  insufficient, problems associated with, 8, 11
  supplements, 54, 98
  types, 97
Fiber Delights, 98
fish and fish oil, 34, 55, 98–99
fish and seafood, risks posed by, 48, 199, 202

flaxseed
  Almond Meal Muffins, 231
  tea from, 155
  versatility of, 149
flaxseed oil, 34, 55, 98–99
Flora-Key, 41, 57–58, 160
Flush step. *See* Week Two
food journal, 142–45
food manufacturing, modern
  antibiotics in food supply, 22, 220
  widespread contamination, 46, 64
food poisoning, 62
foods. *See* Week One; Week Two; Week Three;
    specific types of foods
food sensitivities
  dairy products, 72, 78–80, 84, 134
  delayed responses, 75, 77
  diagnostic questionnaire, 82–83
  elimination diet, 83–84
  versus food allergies, 76–77
  Food Sensitivity Protocol, 83–86
  gluten sensitivity and celiac disease, 8, 75,
    79–82, 222
  growing awareness of, 222
  most common, 84
  risk factors, 77–82
  symptoms, 77
Formula SF 722, 41
Fortify step. *See* Week One
fruits
  avoidance of, 91, 108, 110
  cooked or stewed, 178
  Gut Flush Food Bath, 37
  pantry staples, 135, 136
  raw, 47
  reintroduction into diet, 123–24
  safety during travel, 202
Fuchs, Nan, 94

Galland, Leo, 40
Garbanzo Bean Hummus, 233–34
garlic, 39, 111, 118, 165
genetically modified foods (GMOs), 220
GERD (gastroesophageal reflux disease), 11–13
glutamine, 126–27, 159–60
gluten
  avoidance of, 92
  foods containing, 84
  gluten-free foods, 85
  gluten-free pantry staples, 132, 136,
    137–38
gluten sensitivity and celiac disease
  colon dysfunction from, 8
  growing awareness of, 222
  prevalence of, 81–82
  symptoms and dangers of, 75, 79–81
GMOs (genetically modified foods), 220
Gottschall, Elaine, 109

grains, gluten-free
  breads, 132, 136
  Mega-Grain Quick Bread, 232
  pantry staples, 136, 137–38
  quinoa, 168
groceries
  broths, 135
  canned items, 138–39
  condiments, 138
  cooking and baking ingredients, 138
  dried beans and legumes, 139
  fruits and vegetables, 134–35, 136
  grains and grain products, 136, 137–38
  herbs and spices, 135, 137
  non-dairy milks, 135–36
  nonperishable foods shopping list, 140–41
  oils, 133
  perishables
    Week One, 156–58
    Week Two, 169–71
    Week Three, 182–84
  probiotics, 134
  protein foods, 133, 136–37
  seeds and nuts, 133
  teas, 139
  water, 139–42
  whey protein powders, 139
Gut Flush Food Bath, 37
Gut Flush Plan
  food journal, 142–45, 224
  kitchen preparation, 132–42
  lifelong maintenance, 223–25
  See also protocols; Week One; Week Two; Week
    Three
Gut Grief symptoms, 5

H. pylori, 13, 65–68, 71, 73, 104, 112
HCl (hydrochloric acid)
  HCl Stomach Acid Test, 19
  insufficient, 13, 17
  role of, 16–17
  shortage, disorders associated with, 18
  shortage, signs of, 17–18
  supplements, 27
heartburn, 11–13
heavy metals, limiting exposure to, 198–99
herbs and spices
  Amaranth and Herb-Crusted Chicken, 237–38
  anti-Superbug properties, 72
  cayenne pepper, 72, 111–12, 166
  for flushing, 108–12
  oil of oregano, 40
  pantry staples, 135, 137
  Parsley and Cilantro Pesto, 234
  Parsley Tahini Sauce, 236
  preservative qualities, 122
  storage of, 135
  See also teas

hiatal hernia, 12
high colonics (high enemas), 55, 116–17
home environment
    air fresheners, 219–20
    air quality, 191–93
    bathroom, 194–96
    bedroom, 193–94
    germs, 199–200
    kitchen, 188–91
    laundry room, 197
    pets, 196–97
    shoes, 187–88
hot pepper (cayenne), 111–12, 166
Huggins, Hal, 30
Hummus, Garbanzo Bean, 233–34
hydration, 73, 99–102
hydrochloric acid. *See* HCl (hydrochloric acid)

immune system, 19, 33, 127
indoor air quality, 191–93
insect repellents, 209–10
Inuflora, 98
iodine disinfection of water, 205–6
iron supplements, 7

Jensen, Bernard, 116
journals, 142–45, 224

Kabocha Squash Soup, Creamy, 239–40
kelp, 113
kitchen equipment, 133, 140, 142
kitchen sanitation and safety, 188–91
kitchen staples. *See* groceries

Lactobacillus acidophilus, 20
laundry room environment, 197
laxatives, 7, 9
lead, limiting exposure to, 199
Lemon Caper Dressing, 235
L-glutamine, 126–27, 159–60
licorice, 72–73, 127–28
lifestyle
    constipation and, 7
    exercise, 8, 72, 211, 224
    probiotic depletion and, 24
    yeast overgrowth and, 33–35

main dishes
    Amaranth and Herb-Crusted Chicken, 237–38
    Turkey Meat Loaf Florentine, 238–39
mastic gum, 73
meal plans. *See menu plans*
meats and poultry
    Amaranth and Herb-Crusted Chicken, 237–38
    Black Bean 'n' Beef Chili with a Twist, 242
    kitchen sanitation, 189
    raw and undercooked, 47–48
    safe cooking, 190–91

    Savory Turkey and Swiss Chard Soup, 241
    Turkey Meat Loaf Florentine, 238–39
medications
    antacids, 8, 12–13, 66, 198
    antibiotics, 22–23
    as cause of diarrhea, 8
    encouragement of yeast growth, 39
    laxatives, 7
Mega-Grain Quick Bread, 232
menu plan, Week One
    Fortify strategies, 147–48
    sample menus, 149–55
    shopping list, 156–58
menu plan, Week Two
    addition of supplements, 159–60
    Flush strategies, 160–61
    sample menus, 162–68
    shopping list, 169–71
menu plan, Week Three
    Feeding strategies, 173–74
    as model for lifelong maintenance routine, 172
    sample menus, 175–81
    shopping list, 182–84
menu tips
    almonds, 163
    apple cider vinegar, 179
    artichokes, 155
    avocados, 150
    black beans, 177
    cayenne, 166
    chewing of fibrous foods, 167
    coconut oil, 180
    cooked fruit, 178
    garlic, 165
    ground flaxseed, 149, 155
    herbs, storage of, 135
    Jerusalem artichokes, 152
    kelp powder, 176
    parchment paper, 181
    protein foods, 164
    purslane, 154
    quinoa, 168
    raw vegetables, 162
    refrigeration of leftovers, 151
    sauerkraut, 153
    strawberries, 175
mercury, limiting exposure to, 199
metals, flushing of, 198–99
milk and casein products, 72, 78–80, 84
molasses enemas, 118
mold-containing foods, 92
MRSA (Methicillin-resistant Staphylococcus aureus), 61, 64–65, 115
MSG, 83
mucus production in colon, 6, 10
Muffins, Almond Meal, 231
mugwort, 55, 115–16
multiple vitamins, 41